Healing Addiction with Yoga

A Yoga Program for People in 12-Step Recovery

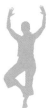

Annalisa Cunningham

FINDHORN PRESS

3rd edition published by Findhorn Press 2010

ISBN 978-1-84409-170-6

Proof read by Michael Hawkins
Inside photographs by Rudy Giscombe,
except pages 66, 123, 124, 137.
Front cover photograph by Candace Jason
Cover design by Thierry Bogliolo
Interior design by Damian Keenan
Printed and bound in China

1 2 3 4 5 6 7 8 9 10 11 12 14 13 12 11 10

Published by
Findhorn Press
305a The Park, Findhorn
Forres IV36 3TE
Scotland, UK

Telephone
+44-(0)1309-690582
Fax
+44-(0)131-777-2177

info@findhornpress.com
www.findhornpress.com

Contents

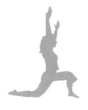

Acknowledgments

There are many people who contributed to the formation of this book. Some I met only briefly during the time I was writing; others are long time friends and family who bless my life with encouragement and support. I value you all.

I would especially like to thank the many yoga students who have participated in my classes as part of their own recovery. Without you, this work would have no purpose. To those of you who shared your journal entries with me, I am especially grateful. Thank you for your confidence. And to those who modeled the poses in the book, I extend a heartfelt thanks. Your energy is so appreciated.

As a student I am forever grateful for the guidance and wealth of information given to me by the yoga teachers I have studied with. Your inspiration has graced my life.

As a person in recovery, I am indebted to all the people in 12-Step program who were there for me when I reached out for help. Thank you for caring.

As an author I appreciate those people who continued to ask for *Stretch & Surrender*, years after it was out of print. Your persistence reminded me that this book has worth.

As a writer I am honored to be working with the people at Findhorn Press and publisher Thierry Bogliolo who's commitment to creating books which offer spiritual inspiration is heart-warming. I would also like to thank Darren Main for his positive recommendation of *Stretch & Surrender* to Findhorn Press, and for writing the foreword. Both Thierry and Darren recognized the value in bringing this book back to life. Thierry came up with the new title and cover, which beautifully displays the essence of healing energy that is the gift of yoga and the 12-Step program.

I'm also grateful to what I call the divine mystery and flow of life which brings continual change, endings and new beginnings, in every step of the journey. *Stretch and Surrender* was published in 1992 and went out of print 6 years later. *Healing Addiction with Yoga* was published in 2003, 11 years after the original book was released. May we all have second chances in life, and may we thrive.

Healing Addiction with Yoga continues to thrive and grow. It is now 17 years after the original book was released. This time the book is being updated with new photos. A warm thanks to Rudy Giscombe who did a fine job with the photography for this edition, and made the project fun. Thanks also to Kirsten Boyd, Amy Briano, Tony Gamboa, Carmel Kennedy, Jasper Lerch, and Patricia Smiley who showed up to model the poses. I'm so fortunate to have such wonderful yoga students and gracious friends. I'd also like to acknowledge and thank Candace Jason who took the cover photo on a fun filled day at the beach near Anchor Bay, California.

Finally, I'd like to give a special acknowledgment to the memory of my Father, Jeff Cunningham, whose life initiated me into a path of searching for wholeness.

Dedication

This book is dedicated to and directed toward people who are following a 12-Step program and attending support meetings such as Alcoholics Anonymous, Narcotics Anonymous, Al-Anon, Nar-Anon, Adult Children of Alcoholics, Overeaters Anonymous, Gamblers Anonymous, Love and Sex addicts Anonymous, and any other meeting which gives support in recovery. Thank you for the risks you are taking in choosing to recover.

I offer this book in appreciation of people involved in recovery and self-discovery; to all people who honor the sacredness of this life, to people who greet others with acceptance, compassion, and forgiveness. You are the people who heal.

Annalisa

The 12-Steps of Alcoholics Anonymous

1.

We admitted we were powerless over alcohol —
that our lives had become unmanageable.

2.

Came to believe that a Power greater than ourselves
could restore us to sanity.

3.

Made a decision to turn our will and our lives over
to the care of God *as we understood Him.*

4.

Made a searching and fearless moral inventory of ourselves.

5.

Admitted to God, to ourselves, and to another human being
the exact nature of our wrongs.

6.

Were entirely ready to have God remove all these defects of character.

7.

Humbly asked Him to remove our shortcomings.

8.

Made a list of all persons we had harmed, and became willing
to make amends to them all.

9.

Made direct amends to such people whenever possible,
except when to do so would injure them or others.

10.

Continued to take personal inventory and when we were wrong
promptly admitted it.

11.

Sought through prayer and meditation to improve our conscious
contact with God as we understood Him, praying only for knowledge
of His will for us and the power to carry that out.

12.

Having had a spiritual awakening as a result of these steps,
we tried to carry this message to alcoholics, and to practice these
principles in all our affairs.

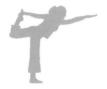

Foreword

In 1935 in the small town of Akron, Ohio, Bill Wilson and Dr. Bob Smith came together to help keep each other sober. Both had been unable to manage their drinking alone, and both knew that their drinking problem was much more than a lack of will or loose morals. Both were on a path that could only lead to "jails, institutions and death."

Through their conversations, they realized that the problem with their drinking was at its core, a spiritual disease. Although their drinking had painfully obvious physical, emotional and psychological consequences, they found that no true healing, and in turn lasting sobriety, could happen until the spiritual nature of their addiction was addressed.

It was out of this realization – the realization of two alcoholics trying to keep each other sober – that Alcoholics Anonymous was born. More importantly, the 12-Steps, which make up the crux of AA Philosophy and recovery, were penned using the work of William Silkworth, MD as a template.

Since those early days with Bill W. and Dr. Bob, a lot has changed. The two became four, and four became many thousands of people. Alcoholics Anonymous has found its way to almost every country on earth. Meetings are held in almost every town and in almost every language. Millions have been able to find freedom from their addiction.

The 12-Steps were not specific to just alcoholics, however. Since the days when Bill W. and Dr. Bob first penned them, scores of 12-Step meetings have sprung up, helping everyone with every form of addiction imaginable. From compulsive over-eaters to gamblers, from co-dependants to sex and love abusers, the 12-Steps have helped millions of people find freedom from their addictions.

Any 12-Stepper will tell you that the secret to the 12-Steps is two-fold. First, it is simple. It is a philosophy that a child could understand. In fact, most children understand the 12-Steps naturally. In a sense the 12-Steps merely remind us of what is encoded in the very cells of our bodies. Rather than burden the recovering person with complex philosophies, the 12-Steps offer a new way of seeing the world and a profoundly effective way of dealing with conflict. In short, the 12-Steps bring order to chaos by teaching the addict to respond to life in ways that are far healthier than feeding one's addiction.

There was a very popular TV show in the 1970s called *The Greatest American Hero*. The basic storyline in the show was about a young man who found a suit. The suit made him a superhero with all sorts of supernatural abilities. The problem was that he didn't have the instruction book to go with it. As a result, the suit was always getting him into trouble. In many ways, addicts are like the Greatest American Hero in that they have tremendous power, and yet they have lost the instructions for how to use it. For many, the 12-Steps are that instruction book.

The second reason the 12-Steps work for so many people is that they are spiritual in nature. Rather than just abstaining from one's addictions, the 12-Steps ask people to fill that void with a deeper understanding of Spirit. Exactly how this is to be done is left up to the individual. But the key to the dramatic success of the 12-Steps is undisputedly their focus on the spiritual.

Addiction is a very multifaceted disease. Although its origin is spiritual, its effects are almost always felt on the physical, emotional and psychological levels as well. It is for this reason that so many people in 12-Step recovery programs find yoga to be an essential tool to support them in their healing.

Like other forms of meditation, yoga addresses the spiritual issues that the 12-Steps would have us address. But it also has notable physical and emotional benefits that are of particular interest to a person in recovery. Annalisa Cunningham's book *Stretch and Surrender (Healing Addictions with Yoga)* is an inspired work that brings these two separate but complementary practices together. The word yoga means "union," and that is exactly what *Stretch and Surrender* achieves. A union of two of the most transformative practices humanity has ever known.

Annalisa's writing is very clear and easy to follow, as are her ideas about using yoga and affirmations with the 12-Steps. Annalisa's words are fluid and easy to wrap your brain around. What is most profound about Stretch and Surrender is the way Annalisa eloquently uses affirmations that sink right to the heart of each pose. The affirmations are obviously richly inspired — channeled even — and they make the connection between body and mind as well as between yoga and the 12-Steps obvious and meaningful.

During my own personal journey through 12-step recovery, and many years of professional observation, I have seen yoga complement the recovery program outlined in the 12-Steps. I have often looked for books to recommend to my students who are in recovery and have not been able to find one—that is until now. *Stretch and Surrender (Healing Addictions with Yoga)* is the bridge between two great spiritual paths that so many in 12-step recovery have been seeking.

Darren John Main,
author of *Yoga and the Path* of the *Urban Mystic*
(www.darrenmain.com)

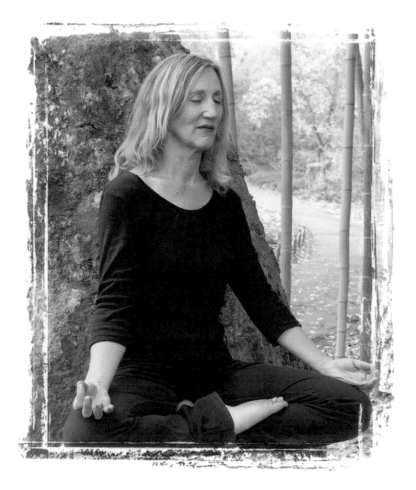

Live and Let Live.

Introduction

Hindsight is a wonderful gift. It reminds us that at any given moment a lot more is going on than we can know. Often the things that happen to us are preparation for the future and for a greater purpose. When I look back on my life I can see that the hardships I've faced have been essential for my growth; the lessons I have learned continue to help me. It was just those hardships that led me to seek healing through yoga, recovery through the 12-Steps, and education in counseling and communication. I realized that putting all those tools together into a single "healing work" is very powerful. This book is my way of sharing this with you.

I began my life growing up in an alcoholic family (and who would ever have thought that I would be forgiving of and even grateful for those hard lessons). By the time I left home at the age of eighteen, I was well prepared as a codependent in denial.

As soon as I was on my own, I immediately became involved in the holistic health field. I now realize that I was subconsciously attempting to heal myself through the study of stress-reduction techniques. I became certified as a massage practitioner and Hatha yoga teacher. Giving massages and teaching yoga were very fulfilling for me. I got my esteem from helping others and I became more relaxed myself. It's true that we teach what we need to learn.

At the same time I was also going to college and studying interpersonal communications. After graduating, I married a man with two children from a previous marriage, and I soon found myself living in another alcoholic family system. The marriage brought out my compulsive, codependent tendencies in full force. I stopped teaching yoga, stopped giving massages, and I put all of my energy into trying to change my husband. As my efforts to change him failed, I became angry, resentful, and depressed. I also developed health problems. After my marriage ended in divorce, a friend suggested that I go to an Al-Anon meeting. There I was introduced to the 12-Step program, which became the foundation for my life. I also began attending Adult Children of Alcoholics meetings.

As I began to get my life back together I accepted a part-time job teaching communications at California State University, Chico. A year later I entered a graduate program in Counseling. I also started teaching yoga again. I continued attending Adult Children of Alcoholic meetings on a regular basis.

The meetings were helping me emotionally and spiritually, but they failed to address the physical aspects of my recovery. For example, after sitting for two hours at a meeting I felt the need to stretch and relax. If I drank a lot of coffee or was bothered by smoke at the meeting, I would end up feeling physically worse than when I had arrived. I was grateful for my knowledge of yoga and relaxation techniques to help me relieve the stress in my body.

My masters program in Counseling led me into an internship at Feather River Alcohol and Chemical Recovery Program in Paradise, California. Three months after volunteering my time there I was offered a job as a counselor. I accepted the position and became more involved in addiction recovery.

One of the first things I discovered while counseling alcoholics and addicts was that they didn't have healthy skills for dealing with stress. When they were stressed they would drink or use. Teaching them new skills for handling stress in their lives seemed like an important ingredient for their continued recovery.

In addition to fulfilling my job requirements as a counselor, I developed a yoga program for both the patients and their family members. I adapted the yoga specifically to the 12-Step philosophy, using affirmations and visualizations designed to encourage and enhance recovery. At first the patients were skeptical. They didn't know what yoga was and were a little afraid to try it. But after one or two sessions the feedback turned positive. The stretching helped people get in touch with their bodies and the relaxation was especially appreciated.

The program was held at a 28 day inpatient recovery hospital. This gave me one month to teach the classes. I offered yoga classes three times a week.

Monday yoga classes were designed for the patients only. Many of these people were going through detox so medical supervision was important. These classes were offered in a slow, gentle manner with emphasis on breathing, visualization, relaxation, and meditation. Postures were done very gently and adapted to each person's ability.

Wednesday yoga classes were available to the family members only. Anyone who lives with an alcoholic or addict is living in a stressful situation. These people also need recovery and are enouraged to attend Al Anon meetings, Codependents Anonymous, Adult Children of Alcoholics, or other 12-Step meetings that are appropriate. In teaching yoga to the family members I emphasized self care and responsibilty since family members have a tendency to blame the addict for their unhappiness. Again the class focus was on gentle, healing yoga with an emphasis on forgiveness, acceptance, honesty and self love.

On Fridays I held the yoga class for both the patients and their family members. This gave them an opportunity to participate in a new activity that they could contine to practice together once the patient returned home. Taking yoga classes together helped establish bonding and a healthy lifestyle change for their continued recovery.

Once the patients were released from the hospital, several people expressed a desire to continue taking my yoga classes. I began offering classes in the general community, structured specifically for people working a 12-Step program. Response was enthusiastic and my classes were full. One of the aspects I appreciated is that my classes attracted people from various branches of the 12-Step movement. A typical class consisted of recovering addicts, alcoholics, codependents, people with eating disorders, and adult children from dysfunctional families. Usually these people are separated with their own special meeting, but in my classes they were gathered together with the common bond of sharing the 12-Step philosophy. Though their problems vary, the solution is the same. In stretching our bodies we also stretch our minds and stretch the limits of our recovery processes.

The 12-Step program of recovery is a physical, mental/emotional, and spiritual program. The practice of yoga is also a physical, mental/emotional and spiritual practice. Both aim at healing the whole person. In my particular situation, however, the spiritual aspect of yoga didn't quite fit. The practice gave me no tools for confronting my codependent issues. On the other hand, I found little support in the 12-Step program for addressing the physical aspects of my disease.

This book synthesizes the best healing aspects of both systems. It offers specific techniques to help the body recover from stress and abuse. It brings the benefits of Hatha Yoga, an Eastern system of health care, into alignment with the Western 12-Step philosophy. This combination opens new doors to recovery. With this book, I invite you to stretch your potential toward wellness and surrender into greater healing.

May you find yoga to be a wonderful support for improved health, relaxation and healing from addiction.

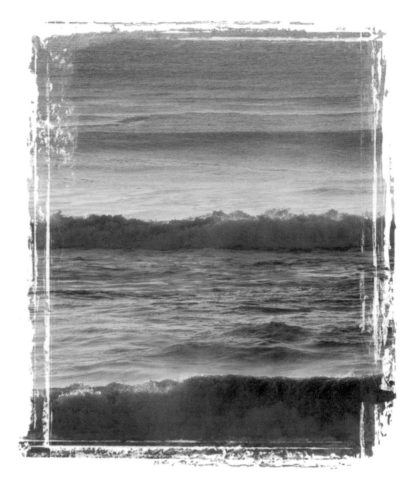

*God grant me the serenity to accept the things
I cannot change, the courage to change the things I can,
and the wisdom to know the difference.*

CHAPTER 1

The 12-Step Approach to Recovery

I was first introduced to the 12-Step program of recovery in 1984. Prior to that time I had explored many of the New Age metaphysical teachings as a way to subconsciously heal myself. In those days, I believed that healing meant transcending my pain. I wanted to skip over my sorrow and unhealed wounds through meditation and other spiritual practices. I used the New Age teachings as a form of denial.

Getting into recovery and meeting people in the 12-Step program gave me a new perspective and depth. It allowed me to plunge into my soul rather than stay in flight of spirit. This was the place where I first explored the unfinished business of my heart.

These days I seek balance. I am not currently involved in the 12-Step programs the way I was when I originally wrote this book. My life has taken me in new directions of nurturing and healing. I do, however, remain in conscious awareness of my need for emotional and spiritual support. I maintain my willingness to grow and change and become all that I can be. Rather than call myself a recovering person, I now refer to myself as someone in discovery. I also no longer readily label myself as codependent or an addict or an adult child of an alcoholic. Beyond those labels, I am a sacred being. Life is sacred and we who are alive are a part of that. I honor my sacredness by continuing to heal and change and grow.

Recovery from alcoholism, substance abuse, and other compulsive, addictive behaviors involves a complete lifestyle change. True recovery means much more than mere sobriety, which is only a beginning. It means recovery of our self-esteem and self worth. It means recovery of our integrity. It means reconnecting with the part of ourselves that is able to give and receive love. It means reconnecting with the mystery of life and with our spirituality. It means recovery of the complete self: physically, mentally, emotionally, and spiritually. True recovery is an ongoing process. It requires a lifestyle that enhances the health and growth of the whole person.

For people who are new to recovery, attending 12-Step meetings can be extremely helpful. I was so grateful to find the support I needed from people at the meetings, and to learn about the 12-Step philosophy which became a foundation for healing in my life. This chapter gives a brief overview of the 12-Steps. I'm including several paragraphs from the original writing of this book which will read as though I am still actively attending 12-Step meetings. Rather than change the sentence structure to past tense I find it more effective to keep my voice alive in the present. As I reread this chapter it helps me honor the path that has lead me to where I am today.

A Person in Recovery

I have called myself a recovering person since the night in 1984 when I attended my first meeting for Adult children of Alcoholics. I refer to myself that way because I attend 12-Step support meetings regularly and I use the steps as a foundation for healing in my life.

When I tell people that I am a recovering person they often ask me what I am recovering from. There is no easy answer to that question. I can explain that I grew up in an alcoholic family and that I am recovering from codependent behaviors, such as trying to change, control, or rescue other people. I may talk about recovering from workaholism, or the period of drug abuse in my life.

Sometimes I simply say that I am recovering from a lack of self love, self-acceptance, self-esteem and self-worth. We all have plenty of things to recover from.

But for me, the more important question is what am I recovering to? When I first got into the 12-Step program I spent a great deal of time looking at the problem. I recognized the fact that I had grown up in an alcoholic family; I analyzed my behaviors and realized how self-defeating they were. With the support of the program I allowed myself to feel the depths of my pain. That was an important process. I needed to move past my denial and accept the problem in order to begin to heal.

Now my focus is on looking at the solution. I am learning new tools and skills to help change my self-defeating patterns, habits, and attitudes. I am choosing a lifestyle that encourages my growth and helps me to love and accept myself exactly as I am right now in recovery: changing, growing, and becoming. The three main pillars of this lifestyle are working the 12-Steps, attending support meetings, and practicing a health care program that takes care of my body, mind, and spirit.

This book is about that kind of health care. It is about finding wellness, finding wholeness in ourselves. It introduces Hatha yoga, an eastern health care system, and adapts it to the 12-Step philosophy to provide a practical how-to guide to improve health and relaxation for recovering alcoholics, addicts, codependents, and adult children from dysfunctional families. It offers new tools for reducing stress and creating healing effects in the body and mind. As you incorporate proper health care into your lifestyle, you will reach new levels of recovery and gain new skills for living in the solution.

I want to emphasize that this health-care system is a practice to be used for recovery along with working the 12-Steps and attending meetings. It is not meant to be a replacement for them. I believe that working the steps can be instrumental in helping people to heal and attain true recovery. The rest of this chapter will briefly describe the steps and will discuss the importance of attending meetings. Those of you who are familiar with this process may want to just skim over these sections and move on to Chapter Two, which explains how Hatha yoga fits into the 12-Steps.

For those of you who are unfamiliar with or new to the 12-Step program, please understand that my explanation is merely a brief introduction. I encourage you to seek out further information about the 12-Step program and to discover for yourself the value and support this program offers. There is a resource list at the end of this book to help you find meetings in your area.

Working the Steps

The 12-Steps, originally designed for Alcoholics Anonymous, have been adapted to help millions of people suffering from dependencies over which they are powerless. The upsurge of fellowships such as Narcotics Anonymous, Overeaters Anonymous, Codependents Anonymous, Sex and Love Addicts Anonymous, and others, attests to the growth and success of the 12-Step movement.

The 12-Steps represent a blueprint for recovery. They constitute a prescription for a spiritual awakening built upon a foundation of fellowship, faith, and service to others. The process entails more than simply stopping the compulsive or addictive behavior. When the addictive behavior is removed from our life, the human condition remains. Being human means experiencing life's sorrows as well as life's joys. We all know that life is not always easy. The 12-Steps offer a framework for self-help in facing life's challenges on life's terms. The most crucial factor in this framework is the acknowledgment and acceptance of the spiritual dimension of our lives.

When we recognize that we are spiritual beings who have forgotten our innate wholeness, our hearts begin to open. As our hearts open, we shift from blame, guilt, and remorse to acceptance, forgiveness, and compassion. We begin to understand that our cravings for alcohol, drugs, and other distractions were attempts to fill a spiritual void. The nature of addiction is to seek ways to connect with something outside the self for a feeling of transcendence and/or worthiness. Unfortunately this outer-directed search often leads to dependency on the object, person, or behavior. Only by embracing our own divine nature can we truly fill the emptiness inside. The 12-Steps, adapted below,* give us a map to a spiritual path and awakening. As we open our hearts and listen within to our own spiritual truth we bring resolution and wholeness into our lives.

The first three steps directly address this spiritual dimension:

STEP ONE
We admit we are powerless over our addiction, that our lives have become unmanageable.

STEP TWO
We believe that a Power greater than ourselves could restore us to sanity.

STEP THREE
We have made a decision to turn our will and our lives to the care of God as we understand Him (or Her or It).

These first three steps have been likened to the experience of the dark night of the soul before the dawn. Often we have to feel hopeless, stuck, and desperate before we are willing to take the first step. The second step shows the promise of light at the end of the tunnel, and the third step leads the way to the light.

After taking these first three essential steps, the remaining nine steps guide us away from self-destructive attitudes and actions to a path of honesty, integrity, forgiveness, and service.

STEP FOUR
We have made a searching and fearless moral inventory of ourselves.

STEP FIVE
We have admitted to God, to ourselves, and to another human being the exact nature of our wrongs.

STEP SIX
We are entirely ready to have God remove all these defects of character.

STEP SEVEN
We humbly ask God to remove our shortcomings.
* For the original language, see page 4.

STEP EIGHT
We have made a list of all persons we have harmed, and are willing to make amends to them all.

STEP NINE
We have made direct amends to such people whenever possible, except when to do so would injure them or others.

STEP TEN
We continue to take personal inventory and when we are wrong, promptly admit it.

STEP ELEVEN
We seek through prayer and meditation to improve our conscious contact with God as we understand Him, praying only for knowledge of His will for us and the power to carry that out.

STEP TWELVE
Having had a spiritual awakening as a result of these steps, we try to carry this message to others, and to practice these principles in all our affairs.

It is important to note that the spirituality emphasized in the 12-Step program is not limited to any specific religion or denomination. Although the word

"God" is used, each person's particular understanding is accepted and encouraged. Oftentimes people in the 12-Step movement substitute the words "Higher Power" to help relay the message that this program is spiritual rather than religious. Spirituality is a universal experience that transcends race, culture, tradition, and belief. It is a feeling that emerges within us when we open our hearts to ourselves, to one another, and to the divine mystery of life. It is a feeling of connection with all living things and a feeling of wholeness that brings healing into our lives.

When I first learned about the 12-Step program and was introduced to the idea of "Higher Power," I related it to the higher energy that I feel when I am in nature. When I spend time in nature, at the ocean for instance, or in the redwoods, I am aware of an energy that is greater than I. The beauty and perfection of nature are miraculous. It is the beauty of nature and the mystery of life that have helped me acknowledge my own divine nature and to surrender my will to the care of a Higher Power.

I don't always feel surrendered though. Sometimes I fall into old ways of thinking; that I am the one in control and that I carry the weight of the world on my shoulders. I start to feel overwhelmed. I forget about my spirituality and I focus on externals to try to get happiness. I lose connection with the higher energy. I start to feel defeat and lack in myself. Then I have to remind myself to go back to the first step, and admit that I am powerless, that my life has become unmanageable. From there I go right on to the second step: there is a power greater than myself that can restore me to sanity. And so I surrender (step three) — over and over again. It is a continual process — this is "working the steps." Each step can be done over and over again as we slowly peel away the layers of our self-defeating attitudes and behaviors. Each step has a gift to offer.

In the fourth step we are asked to make an inventory of ourselves. This requires self-honesty and a willingness to look at ourselves for who we are and where we've been. Self-honesty is necessary for building self-respect. In working this step, our capacity to grow into who we can become is strengthened.

Step five encourages us to admit the nature of our wrongs to God, to ourselves, and to another person. When we discuss our human mistakes and failures with another person, we acquire enough humility and honesty to truly heal. This undertaking places us in a vulnerable position, yet it gives us a feeling of relief as we accept our mistakes and become eligible for forgiveness.

The sixth step signifies that we are ready to change. For many of us, this first requires that we realize we are worthy of healing. Every one of us — everyone who has life — is worthy of healing, but many of us who are recovering from self-destructive attitudes and behaviors have trouble believing that. Regaining a sense of self-worth is an important part of recovery.

In step seven we turn to God and ask Him (or Her or It) to remove our shortcomings. This is an action toward accepting our worth, and our right as a human being to heal and to be whole.

Step eight encourages us to make a list of all the people we have harmed and become willing to make amends to them. This is hard work. It requires honesty and strength, yet gives us a new way of relating to others and to ourselves. It indicates a willingness to swallow our own stubborn pride in exchange for restoring truth and respect, which are essential for healthy relationships.

In step nine we make amends, whenever possible, to people we have harmed. Working this step helps us repair our relationships with others, and allows us to free ourselves from guilt. It helps us regain a clear conscience and a peaceful mind.

Step ten asks us to continue to take our personal inventory, generally on a daily basis, so we learn to admit our wrongs when they occur, knowing that to be human is to make mistakes. This step offers us the gift of integrity as we develop the strength to be honest at all times with others and with ourselves.

The eleventh step gives us tools for deepening our connection with our Higher Power and helps us remember our own divine nature. It allows us to maintain a feeling of serenity in our lives.

In the twelfth step, having experienced a healing and a spiritual awakening as a result of these steps, we are encouraged to use these principals in every part of our lives and to share them with others. This step reminds us that recovery is an ongoing process. We remain humble as we keep working the steps as guidelines in our daily lives, and offer them in service to others.

The 12-Steps are guideposts. They point the way to a life with meaning. Without faith our lives are a meaningless succession of unrelated events and chance happenings. We hope for the best and fear the worst. When we are faced with failure and defeat we feel lost and empty. Our souls have nowhere to turn.

When we surrender our lives to the care of a Higher Power we get in harmony with the divine nature of all living things. Our souls can rest in faith, knowing that there is a spiritual presence guiding our lives. This puts our problems and difficulties into perspective. Rather than worrying and fretting over our present circumstances, we begin to trust this process called living. We awaken to the inner knowing that life is sacred. We are sacred. Acknowledging our spirituality gives our lives purpose and meaning.

In addition to opening us up to our spirituality, the steps help us to open our hearts to ourselves. We get in touch with the child within who can lead us to our true innocence. The 12-Step program helps us to remember that we are all children of God.

The 12-Step program is not for everyone — there are many paths to healing and finding wholeness — but for those who need it, want it and are ready to begin a lifelong process of spiritual and emotional development, it can be wonderful. Attending a meeting is one step in that process, usually the first.

Attending Meetings

"Hi. My name is Annalisa and I am a sacred being who is capable of healing, growing, changing, and becoming all that I can be."

Going to support meetings is the basic building block to working a 12-Step program. Numerous groups, patterned after Alcoholics Anonymous, have been formed to offer help and support to people who are suffering from compulsive and addictive behaviors. Regardless of what type of addiction or problem the group members are struggling with, the meetings provide a support system for recovery, using the 12-Steps as a framework.

These groups are extremely helpful because each member in the group is experiencing the same problem. We can relate to each other with true understanding and compassion. Knowing that you are not alone with your problem is in itself a relief. The groups provide a supportive environment where people can talk about their experiences without being judged or criticized. People are free to share whatever they want with the group. Anonymity is required; only first names are exchanged, and whatever is spoken in that room stays there.

Talking is not a requirement, it's entirely acceptable to choose not to talk, and just be there to listen. In fact, learning to listen is an important part of the meetings. When somebody is talking, no crosstalk is allowed. The person who speaks is given the respect of everyone's full attention, without interruptions. Have you ever been given the opportunity to say whatever you want without being interrupted or cut off? It's a rare and special gift.

Gifts are gained from listening to others as well. It is a special feeling to be with people who talk openly about their pain and failures, as well as their joys and virtues. So often in our daily lives we are taught to pretend that everything is fine, even when it's not.

At 12-Step meetings there is no pretending. If someone is feeling angry or sad or fearful about a situation in his or her life, that person may openly reveal these feeling. Other people may talk about the mistakes they've made and the hurt they feel.

At first it can be a little startling to hear people be so honest. We're all used to hiding behind addiction and masks that help us avoid our true feelings. Yet getting in touch with our feelings and learning to express them are important parts of our recovery. Attending meetings means placing yourself in an environment of honest and caring interaction

When I first got into the 12-Step program I went to lots of meetings. These days I don't go as often, but I know they are there if I need one. I think it is very special to know that there is a place where people who need support can go. No one is excluded from the 12-Step program; anyone who wants to be there can be, and the meetings are cost free. Meetings can differ with the people who attend them; it's a good idea to check out several to find a group you are comfortable with.

I've sometimes heard people outside the program say that attending meetings becomes another obsession or addiction. When I hear this, I have to smile within, because these people have no idea of what a wonderful fellowship they are missing out on. Because of the 12-Step way of life, recovering people are some of the most humble, honest, and supportive people I've ever met. This is not to say that they have no flaws. They are openly human, flaws and all.

At the meetings we are taught to give to others by being open and honest about our own lives and by listening with our full attention and compassion as others speak about theirs. This exchange within the group is extremely healing.

It is ironic that those of us who follow the 12-Step way of life wouldn't have attended our first meeting if we hadn't been faced with overwhelming problems and unbearable pain. What began as a curse has become a blessing in disguise. Our problems brought us to this fellowship and to a new faith in life with the 12-Step path as our guide.

Ultimately the process becomes a lifestyle that enhances the development of our well-being. As we choose to recover we learn new ways of living. We learn to treat ourselves as a friend and to enjoy the possibilities for growth and positive change that life offers.

Journal Entry

I think the thing that impresses me most about the 12-Step meetings is the amount of humor people in recovery have. Once I got past the initial denial and pain, I found my sense of humor returned with a vengeance.

I've found through the years that once you let go of things, and treat them as a learning experience, you can laugh at how much energy you wasted in anger and frustration

I still get annoyed or angry about things, but by the time I get into bed at night it has dwindled down to a petty inconvenience, and I let it go because tomorrow is always a new, exciting day.

The 12-Step program has helped me develop this attitude of letting go. It has given me a sense of peace and hope in my life.

Kat *(Recovering Addict)*

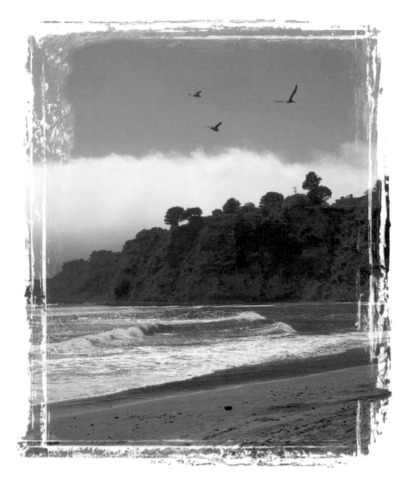

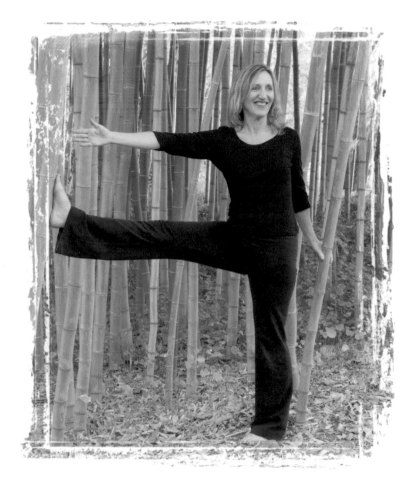

Let go and let God.

CHAPTER 2

How does Yoga fit in with the 12-Steps?

I discovered Hatha yoga long before I got into a 12-Step program of recovery. I wanted to learn about yoga because I was in the business of reducing stress. I earned my living by giving massages.

Every day people came to me complaining of tight shoulders, stiff necks, aching backs, and sore muscles. I used my massage techniques to work the tension out of muscles, relieve tightness, and relax the person completely. A typical client came in feeling uptight from life's pressures, and left feeling calm and relaxed. But just a week or two later the same person would call me up again desperately wanting another massage. I loved the job; I felt needed.

My practice grew and soon I was overwhelmed; I could only give so many massages in one day! I began thinking to myself that there must be something these people could do for themselves to help relieve the stress and tension they felt.

That's when I decided to study Hatha yoga. I had heard that yoga is a form of stretching exercise used for relieving stress and tension; I thought yoga might offer techniques for relaxing the person when massage wasn't available. I wanted to learn yoga as a form of self-massage I could teach to my clients.

It was through the study of yoga that I first learned about healing the complete self: physically, mentally, emotionally, and spiritually. The methods used in Hatha yoga work to improve physical health and well-being, increase mental concentration and clarity, balance and calm the emotions and, through meditation, enable one to come closer to the realization of his or her own spiritual nature.

After one month of practicing Hatha yoga on a regular basis I began to notice positive changes in my own well-being. I felt better physically, calmer emotionally, clearer mentally, and I began to acknowledge the feeling of a spiritual presence in my life.

The spiritual presence, however, was the most difficult for me to define. I didn't have a God or a guru I believed in and followed, like many of the people

I studied yoga with seemed to have. I had no desire to worship or follow some-one else's teachings. I admitted that I was aware of a spiritual presence in my life but I was uncomfortable with labeling that presence and I had no desire to surrender my will. I still felt that I was in control of life and managing things quite nicely. That feeling persisted until I got married. I married a charming, attractive man who had problems with alcohol and with being honest. I wanted to change him, but of course I couldn't. As time went on things got worse. My husband refused to go to counseling. I was at a loss of what to do.

The ending of my marriage was the catalyst that brought me to the 12-Step program. By the time I got there I had stopped doing yoga completely, as well as other activities that were nurturing for me. My health had deteriorated alarm-ingly. I was physically sick, emotionally depressed, mentally fatigued, and spiri-tually empty. It was difficult to admit that I was powerless and that my life had become unmanageable.

One of the first things I heard when I got into recovery was the importance of healing the complete self. I was told that addiction is a threefold disease: physical, mental/emotional, and spiritual. This made sense to me because of my experience with Hatha yoga. I had already learned how the different aspects of myself affected one another. If a situation makes me feel bad emotionally, then I have less energy physically. Any physical pain will disturb my mental outlook on life. When I am in touch with my spirituality, I feel better emotion-ally. When I feel good physically, it is easier to meditate, which helps me get in touch with my spiritual self. All these aspects are interrelated. If we ignore any one aspect, the rest suffer.

One of the greatest gifts the 12-Step program gave me was a comfortable outlet for and expression of my spirituality. I liked the idea of a Higher Power as I under-stood it. As I began working the steps and going to meetings I became willing to surrender to my Higher Power. The emotional support I received at the meetings was wonderful. I was able to openly share my feelings and I felt appreciated. The understanding and clarity I gained from the program were also very healing.

The only aspect I didn't find specific help for in the 12-Step program was the physical. The program offered me no tools for healing my physical self. This was especially important for me then, because the emotional stresses of my codependent marriage and the painful process of divorce had seriously affected my health. Simply put, I was stressed out. I was nervous and seldom ate. I had lost so much weight that I looked like a skeleton. My muscles were always tense and my neck and shoulders hurt. I had also developed insomnia and had been taking sleeping pills for several months.

Fortunately, I had already learned the skills for healing my physical self from my study of Hatha yoga. When I got into 12-Step recovery I also started practicing Hatha yoga again, the way I used to before I was married. Hatha yoga complemented my recovery work perfectly. It helped my body to heal, my mind to clear, and my emotions to calm. It allowed me quiet time each day to reflect upon my own spiritually.

As time went on I began incorporating the 12-Step philosophy into my yoga practice. While I was stretching my body I thought about the positive sayings I learned at the meetings, such as "easy does it" or "let go and let God." I started making up my own affirmations which helped me with self-esteem, and I said them to myself while I held the yoga poses. When I finished stretching my body I took some quiet time to relax and I prayed to my Higher Power. I ended by meditating and I came out of the entire process with a feeling of serenity.

Since that time the practice has expanded. I now teach classes to other recovering people. I have assigned a positive thought or affirmation to each yoga posture that correlates to the 12-Steps. The visualizations I use for relaxation are deliberately intended to encourage recovery. The classes are designed to reduce stress and tension while increasing self-worth and self-esteem. Learning to take care of my body is an important ingredient in my recovery. Hatha yoga stretches and relaxes the body, calms the mind, and helps the body recover from stress and abuse. It is self-constructive rather than self-destructive behavior. In addition to attending meetings and working the 12-Steps, I practice Hatha yoga as part of my recovering lifestyle.

What Is Hatha Yoga?

Yoga is a system of exercise, breathing, and meditation developed thousands of years ago in India. It is the world's oldest system of personal growth, encompassing body, mind, and spirit. The goal of yoga practice is the total harmony between body, mind, and spirit in each individual and, even further, a union between the individual and the divine.

The ancient yogis understood the interrelationship between the body, mind, and spirit and the need for balance and health in all three areas as a foundation for personal spiritual awakening. Thus they developed a system for maintaining this balance, a system that addressed body, breath, mind, social and moral behavior, and spiritual exercises.

Hatha yoga is the branch of yoga that deals with the physical body. It is a system that combines stretching, breathing, positive thinking, relaxation, meditation, and a healthy diet to create a practical method for improving health – and for developing a foundation for a deeper understanding as well. The system of Hatha yoga can be thought of as the owner's manual for a human body. Just as the owner's manual for an automobile tells you how to take care of your car, Hatha yoga gives you guidelines for taking care of your body. A car requires regular upkeep to keep it running properly. The human body is no different.

Your Body is the Vehicle that Houses Your Soul

Sometimes I think that people take better care of their cars than they do of their bodies. They keep their cars clean, well fueled, lubricated, and in good working condition. Think about it. What do you do when your car gives you a warning that something is wrong? Let us say that you are driving down the road and you notice the brake warning light on your dashboard has come on. You check to make sure you have not left the emergency brake on. You try the brakes to make sure they still work. The chances are good that you will pull into a service station to talk to a mechanic. If he discovers you are out of brake fluid, you gladly put more in. People want their cars to run well because they are dependent on them to go places. Your car does a lot for you, but what about your body? If you wear out your body, where are you going to live?

Most people in recovery have a history of disregarding their bodies. Whether from years of substance abuse or simply from holding in pent-up feeling and tensions, the body accumulates stress. Stress in the body lowers our energy and physical vitality.

Fatigue is one of our bodies' first warning signs that we are out of balance in our lives. If we pay attention to this sign and allow ourselves some rest and relaxation, we can face whatever situation we are in with a clearer mind. But so often people ignore this signal. For instance, many times in my life when I felt fatigued I drank coffee so I would not notice how tired I felt.

There are many ways to mask and ignore the body's signals, but in the long run we are only doing harm to ourselves. When we ignore the small signals of the tension that is held in our bodies, we accumulate stress. Prolonged or chronic stress can result in various problems, such as migraine headaches, ulcers, backaches, high blood pressure, insomnia, breathing problems, digestive disorders, skin problems, depression, and disease. The continued use of alcohol and drugs on top of stress puts an additional toll on the body. Deterioration of organs (heart and liver), hormonal imbalance, and malnutrition are common ailments of alcoholics and addicts.

Often it takes a severe health problem to scare people enough to reach out for help. We can only hope that by the time they get the help they need they have not done irreversible damage to their bodies. But luckily, the human body has a miraculous ability to heal. I have been amazed at how much abuse the body can take and then turn around and heal itself given the opportunity with proper care.

Hatha yoga offers a formula for giving the body proper care. A healthy diet, breathing exercises, stretching, relaxation, meditation, and positive thinking are the ingredients of this formula. Practicing Hatha yoga helps the body heal and keeps it running properly. It is not just a formula of exercise like calisthenics or aerobics. It is a formula which honors the larger spiritual quest as well. The word yoga means "union". For me, practicing Hatha yoga brings a strengthened sense of union with my Higher Power. It is a practice that heals my body, quiets my mind, and gives me a feeling of serenity.

How Does Hatha Yoga Heal the Body?

There are many physiological benefits to practicing Hatha yoga. Almost immediately your body responds positively to deep breathing and stretching. You begin to relax. As you stretch your muscles, you are lengthening them. Longer muscles are more efficient and less prone to injury. The postures help you to become flexible and strong. Your internal organs are toned as well. As you continue to practice the poses, they help flush toxins out of your body by activating and stimulating circulation, digestion, and elimination. Regular practice also helps to regulate your metabolism and the working of all the glands and organs as well as the nervous system and the mind.

The breathing exercises help to increase your lung capacity. This allows you to bring more oxygen into your body to nourish your cells. Deep, full breathing also works to calm your emotions and lower your stress level.

The deep relaxation at the end of each yoga session quiets your mind, slows your pulse, and brings your body to a state that is receptive to healing. This allows for the total rejuvenation of your body and mind, as all fatigue vanishes.

A healthy diet promotes nutritional food that contains all the necessary vitamins, minerals, amino acids, and enzymes needed to help your body heal and rebuild. Positive thinking creates an attitude of respect and self-acceptance toward your body so that you take better care of it, as well as other aspects of yourself. And lastly, meditation allows for a feeling of tranquility and serenity that carries into all aspects of your life.

Journal Entry

I have been sober for approximately 19 months. I have always been very tense and carry a great deal of stress throughout my body. In the past I had heard about yoga's therapeutic benefits and was interested in giving it a try. I was introduced to yoga through Annalisa's class about seven months ago. Shortly after beginning the class, I started doing yoga on a daily basis in the mornings after waking up.

Not long after I started practicing yoga, my body began to become more flexible, releasing a great deal of the tension that I accumulate on a daily basis. Along with the physical relaxation I have experienced a similar "calming" of my mind. I feel that yoga has helped me to become more centered spiritually and emotionally.

Yoga is an important part of my recovery today. It is an excellent maintenance program for relieving stress and achieving some peace of mind on a daily basis. It enables me to get in touch with myself and become more aware of my body. The more I practice, the greater the benefits I receive. I was hesitant and skeptical when I began yoga, but today I can say with confidence, "When I stretch my body I stretch my soul."

Steve *(Recovering Alcoholic, ACoA)*

Journal Entry

The hardest part of a successful recovery program for me has been incorporating healthy coping mechanisms in my life. I wanted a healthy way to relieve stress without using my old habits. Hatha yoga is becoming a very important part of my recovery program. The positive affirmations we focus on while stretching are really great.

I am learning to replace all the negative messages instilled in my head since childhood with positive ones. Messages such as being at peace with myself, forgiveness, and surrender. Gentleness, being loved, self-acceptance, honesty, and my dependence on a higher power are all new and wonderful ways of thinking. The more I say these things, the freer I feel from the addict in me.

Physically, Hatha yoga is helping me become in tune with my body. For the first time in my life I am learning how to relax. Through gentle stretching and meditation I am able to relieve stress. I have become more flexible. I am learning how to be aware of my breathing patterns. When I breathe deep and easy, my mind and body relax. I am not so uptight. I like myself better.

Candice *(Recovering Addict/Alcoholic)*

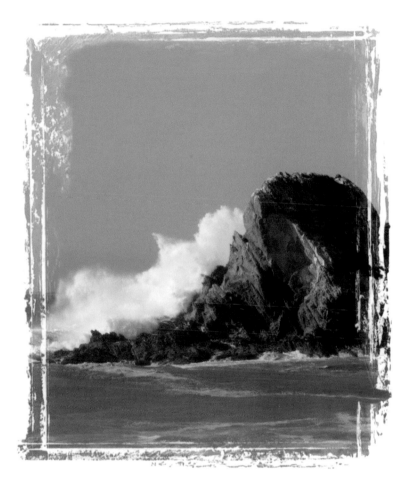

One day at a time.

CHAPTER 3

Tools for
Choosing to Live

W hen I was eighteen I had a friend who was in her forties — and much
younger than I. I say this because she was in touch with her inner child.
I was not. I remember hiking a mountain with her one day. My body was out
of shape and she climbed easily ahead of me. I was only halfway up when she
reached the top. I looked up at her and heard her shout to the universe: "Life is
beautiful. I am alive".

I didn't feel that way at all. I was depressed over my father's recent death. I
was living in a college dormitory, which I hated. I was overweight and out of
touch with my feelings. In many ways I was numb.

Recovery is about choosing to become un-numbed. It is about making
the choice to live — to really live. Everyone alive is breathing, but most
people are not breathing fully. They are not feeling fully. Denial of feelings is a way to deny life. Negative thinking and self-criticism are ways to
negate life. The excessive use of alcohol, drugs, and food are methods for
numbing life.

The decision to embrace life can be the start of a scary process, as we
allow ourselves to feel life's pain as well as life's joy. During this process of
unnumbing is is important for us to have compassion for ourselves. AA
meetings offer support from others who understand the process we are going through in recovery. The 12-Steps and the meeting are powerful tools
for recovery. In addition to participating in a 12-Step program, it is helpful
to learn and incorporate new habits and skills that are self-nurturing and
reinforce our choice to live. Yoga teaches specific techniques that aid in our
process of healing and enhance our feeling of aliveness. The tools offered
in this book incorporate my knowledge and experience in yoga as well as in
counseling. In this chapter, we will be talking about: breathing techniques,
positive affirmation, journal writing, and attitude.

Choosing to Breathe

Breathing is the essence of yoga. It is also the essence of our life. Breath is our life force. As long as we breathe, we are alive. We can go for days without sleep, food, and water, but we can live for only mere minutes without breathing. Human life begins with our first breath and ends with our last. What happens in the passage between these two breaths reveals the quality of the life we have lived.

For those of us who are recovering from addiction and self-destructive behavior, the decision to learn to breathe more fully is the decision to take in life more fully and to choose health over illness. Proper breathing is intrinsically linked with relaxation, with the emotions, and with the health of the body itself.

When we are tense, we have a tendency to hold our breath or to take rapid and shallow breaths. When we are depressed or emotionally upset, our breathing becomes uneven. If we are frightened, we may gasp or hold our breath. When we are angry, our breathing becomes rapid and choppy.

On the other hand, when we are relaxed, our breathing becomes slow and even. The more deeply and slowly we breathe, the more we nurture and relax our entire body. Complete breathing oxygenates the blood, which in turn feeds the organ systems in the body. As you learn to breathe slowly and deeply, you will calm your mind and quiet your emotions. You cannot remain worried and upset for long if you are breathing in a calm and controlled manner. Deep breathing is a tool for getting a handle on your emotions, calming your mind, and relieving your body of tension.

Then, with a calm, clear mind, you will have the strength to face the situation in front of you — however tough it may be.

If you are like most people, you probably live your life without paying attention to the way you are breathing. Unless you suffer from asthma, emphysema, or some other breathing impairment, your breathing is more or less an automatic process. Yet the breathing process lends itself easily to conscious control. With practice you can learn to breathe deeply and fully so that you get the highest benefit from each breath you take.

One of the easiest ways to learn to breathe fully is to practice while lying down on your back. I like to practice the following diaphragmatic breathing exercise just before I go to sleep. It is especially helpful if I have a lot on my mind and am having trouble getting to sleep. As I focus my mind on my breathing, I let go of my thoughts, my body relaxes, and I drift off into the Land of Nod.

Diaphragmatic Breathing

Lie down on your back and place your right hand on your lower abdomen. As you inhale slowly, think of bringing the air all the way down to the lower abdomen so that your stomach expands with the incoming air. If your hand is resting on your stomach, you will feel it rising with the incoming air.

As you slowly exhale, you will feel your hand lowering and your stomach hollowing with the release of air. Continue breathing slowly and deeply until you have completed ten breath cycles. You should be breathing through your nose while you do this exercise. Practice this technique as often as possible so that it becomes easy for you to do.

Once you feel comfortable with breathing deeply while lying on your back, you can begin to incorporate deep breathing into your daily life. Practice the following Complete Breath exercise while sitting or standing, at any time during your day.

The Complete Breath

Begin by inhaling the air all the way down to your lower abdomen so that your stomach and lower back expand with the incoming air. Continue bringing air in so that your rib cage expands, and finalize the inhalation with an expansion of your chest so that your collarbones rise slightly. With this complete breath your entire torso is filled with oxygen, which helps nourish and relax all the muscles and cells in your body. Exhale slowly in the same manner. Begin by releasing the air in your chest, then releasing the air in your rib cage, and finally emptying your abdomen so that your stomach hollows with the release of breath.

You may have noticed that there are three body parts in the complete breath. A good way to practice experiencing the breath in your body is to place your hands on each part while you are breathing.

Begin by placing your hands on your abdomen as you practice several complete breaths. Breathe through your nose and feel the belly expand with the inhalation, like a balloon filling up with air. As you exhale you feel the belly gently hollow.

Next, place your palms on the sides of your ribs with your fingers coming around to the front. Feel the ribs expanding with every inhalation and gently contracting with every exhalation. Bring the air all the way into your abdomen and continue bringing air into the rib cage, where your hands are now.

Finally, place your hands on your chest with your fingers resting on your collarbones. Feel the chest and collarbones gently rise as you complete the inhalation and gently fall as you begin the exhalation. The entire torso moves in rhythm with the breath, fully expanding and slowly contracting, gently and naturally.

With practice you will be able to breathe this way smoothly and continuously. It may be difficult at first because it's different from what you are used to, but keep in mind that you are developing healthier habits for your recovery. Remember that the deeper and slower you breathe the more relaxed you will be. It is a simple change to make and yet can help so much in reducing stress.

Positive Thinking

Another way to reduce stress is to develop the habit of positive thinking. As you breathe in nurturing oxygen, use your thoughts to nurture yourself as well. Thinking positively can help develop a healthy self-esteem. Thinking negatively can create a poor self-image and actually create tension in the body.

In AA they have a saying for thinking negatively about yourself, others, and life in general. It is called "stinkin' thinkin'". Stinkin' thinkin' includes criticism, blame, worry, and judgment. It is limiting because it is the opposite of acceptance, responsibility, trust, and love.

When I first began practicing Hatha yoga I would often catch myself falling into the stinkin' thinkin' trap. While holding a pose, my mind would wander and I'd use the time to dwell on my problems, or on uncompleted projects I needed to get done, or on the weight I wanted to lose. I also criticized myself because I wasn't flexible. Even though I was helping my body by stretching, I was beating up on myself with my thoughts.

Since that time I have assigned a positive affirmation to each yoga posture. I say the affirmation silently to myself while holding the pose. This combination of positive thinking with the postures is extremely powerful. You are sending an emphatic message to your own mind and emotions that those old ways of stinkin' thinkin' no longer control you. At the same time, the affirmations improve the quality of the pose by reminding you of the real purpose of the exercise. For instance, while doing the Camel Pose, which requires lifting up the breastbone and opening the chest as you arch back, I use the affirmation "I am open and receptive to life's lessons." Thus, the opening and healing are achieved on three levels simultaneously as I physically demonstrate, mentally affirm, and spiritually acknowledge my receptivity to the lessons in my life. This integration allows learning to take place on a deeper level within. It allows me to fully benefit from the interconnections between my physical, mental/emotional, and spiritual self.

Our bodies respond to our inner messages. When we hold onto thoughts of worry and fear, our bodies respond with tension. When we criticize ourselves with thoughts of judgment, our bodies respond with tension. With negative thinking we lower our immune system along with our self-esteem. When we begin to change our thinking from negative to positive, we are nurturing ourselves.

I found that making up affirmations to hold in my mind while I am holding the yoga postures was very helpful. I like to think of my yoga practice as a time to wash away all negative thinking, all worry and fret, and to allow my mind to focus on the positive. Each affirmation is attuned to the inner feeling of the pose and helps develop self-worth. Now when I teach yoga to other recovering people, I always use affirmations.

Sometimes new students feel a little foolish at first if I ask them to repeat an affirmation with me. They are not used to verbalizing self-affirming statements. When this happens, I gently encourage people to silently repeat the affirmation to themselves. Even a few minutes of a self-affirming thought can be healing. Affirmations teach us to think positively and to open our minds to loving and accepting ourselves.

Thinking positively does not mean ignoring problems or pretending they are not there. Using affirmations in that way would be like putting whipped cream on garbage. There is a time to face the parts of ourselves we may not like, to grieve, and to be sad. AA meetings are designed as a place to express our feelings, whatever they are. By going to meetings and working the 12-Steps we can learn the difference between genuinely expressing negative feelings and letting them go, or falling into a stinkin' thinkin' pattern where we hold onto a negative attitude toward life.

Learning to change my pattern of stinkin' thinkin' took effort on my part. I began to notice how often I was critical of myself. I made a conscious effort to say something positive each time I caught myself judging in a negative way. I was shocked to realize how often I put myself down. Think about your own patterns of "self-talk": are you a good friend to yourself or are you your own harshest critic? If you find yourself dwelling on the negative, deepen your breathing to interrupt a negative thought. Then replace it with something positive. The use of affirmations, not only in your yoga practice, but throughout your day, can make a profound difference in your inner and outer environments.

Journal Writing

When I first got into recovery and learned how growing up in an alcoholic family had affected me, I felt like a volcano had erupted inside me: the hot lava of anger, sadness, and grief just kept pouring out of me.

It was during that time I started keeping a journal, and I've been writing in one ever since. Writing down my feelings has helped me to discover parts of myself I wasn't aware of. I dialogued with my inner child and discovered how scared and unprotected the child within me felt. I dialogued with my inner parent who was often saying, "I should do this. I should do that." And I realized that my inner parent created a lot of guilt. I dialogued with the grown-up in me who wanted to learn a balance between play and responsibility. As I wrote I began to notice patterns in my life – patterns in the way I reacted to certain situations. I saw patterns in my behavior towards others. I saw patterns in my thoughts. Writing was very revealing.

Journal writing is an invaluable tool for deepening our relationship with ourselves. Because it was (and is) so helpful in my own recovery I began to include journal writing in my yoga practice. After stretching, relaxation, and meditation I get out my journal and write. I've found that taking time for journal writing immediately after practicing Hatha yoga and meditation is ideal because I am relaxed, I have quieted my being, and I am more in touch with my intuitive self. I write about feelings that come up in my daily life. I write about recovery issues that come up — such as my fear of intimacy or my lack of self-esteem. I note my reactions and I notice my progress.

I've developed an entire list of writing exercises whose themes are around recovery issues. I usually introduce these into the yoga classes I teach for recovering people.

You can do this yourself. For example, take the theme of forgiveness. Think about the people in your life that you need to forgive. Make a list of these people. Write about how each person hurt you and how angry or disappointed that made you feel. Try dialoguing with each person, telling them how you feel about what happened between you. As you are writing notice if there is any resentment within yourself that you carry toward these people. See if you can let the resentment go. If you're not ready to forgive yet, that's okay. Work with it. Notice if you need to forgive yourself for anything. Write about it. There is no right or wrong way to keep a journal. Just start writing. You'll be surprised at what things come out on paper when you start writing. Journal writing becomes a creative process.

Sometimes I write with my less dominant left hand which is more difficult for me and makes me feel vulnerable. Through my own process of recovery I've come to understand that vulnerability is a strength. I used to think of it as a weakness and I would pretend that everything was all right even if inside I didn't feel it was. Now when I feel vulnerable, angry, scared, or even unsure of what I'm feeling, rather than cover it up I start writing in my journal and this helps me to get in touch with my feelings and to understand myself better. It helps me to be more compassionate with myself. Nobody reads my journal. It is confidential. This is a matter of personal choice. For me it represents the trust I have with myself — I can confide in myself.

Journal writing teaches self-expression and acceptance. It helps us to become more conscious of our innermost thoughts and feelings. Journaling immediately after practicing Hatha yoga and meditation is ideal because these practices enable us to experience a state of peace and receptivity. Personal insights flow. Divine, intuitive guidance is received. The pen records our God-given thoughts with clarity and ease.

Sample Journal Writing Exercise

LETTING GO
List the things, situations, and people in your life that you are having a difficult time letting go of. Write down what you like about your life right now and what you don't like. What can you add to your life to enrich and strengthen it?

Attitude: Willingness and Patience

You need two ingredients to practice Hatha yoga: willingness and patience. First you need to be willing to set time aside for your yoga practice. Keep in mind that this is a self-constructive behavior. You are worth the time and effort it requires! Have you ever not wanted to go to an AA meeting because you just didn't feel like going through the effort to get there, yet once you got there you were glad you went? I've found yoga to be the same way. I always feel better after I've done my yoga. I suggest twenty minutes a day to start. The same time each day is best: consistency becomes habit. I usually practice in the morning because it starts my day with a positive feeling of well-being. Some people prefer evenings so that they can unwind from the day. The most important time is when you will be free from interruptions. For some people, this may sound impossible. Our busy lives leave little room for ourselves; work, children, phone calls, emails, and household responsibilities fill our waking hours. Taking time out to nurture ourselves seems like too much of a luxury. And yet those of us who don't take time out for self-nurturing are more likely to relapse into self-destructive behavior due to stress. The willingness to slow down and relax is essential to our overall well-being. With this in mind, yoga practice becomes an exercise in affirming your self-worth. Even if you start out stretching only 10 minutes a day, you are still taking little steps in learning self-care and relaxation. To help you do this I have provided suggested daily postures at the end of chapter 4 that let you start out slowly and gently, ten to twenty minutes a day. For those of us who have been self-destructive in our past, learning to take care of ourselves and to realize our worthiness is essential to our recovery. So be willing to give yourself this time.

The second important quality is patience. In my life I have had a difficult time being patient. My tendency in life is, "I want it and I want it now." This tendency to be impatient has caused me some heartache as I have been impulsive and demanding.

When I got into recovery, patience was such an important quality for me to learn that one day I bought some poster paper, painted the word PATIENCE on it in huge letters, and hung it on the wall facing my bed. Every morning the first thing I saw when I woke up was the word PATIENCE. Every night the last thing I saw before I went to sleep was the word PATIENCE. I kept the poster up for three months. It was an effective reminder.

Patience is an important attribute to have while practicing Hatha yoga. When practicing the postures you need to be patient with your body. Never strain or force a stretch. Stretch gently, going to the point of comfort and only slightly beyond that point, slowly, easily. Yoga should never hurt. "Easy does it" is a good motto here. The goal is not to see how far you can stretch, but rather to work with your body in helping it to open and relax at its own rate of surrender. If you force a stretch beyond your body's limit, you will hurt yourself.

Learn to listen to your body. Pay attention to your body, and become aware of how your body is feeling and what messages your body is sending you. If your body feels especially tight or tense, acknowledge that feeling and move very slowly. If you move slowly, you will know when you have reached your limit. Never push past your limit; stretch slowly only to the edge of your maximum stretch. You should be able to feel the stretch, but it should not be painful. Hold the pose at that edge and breathe slowly and deeply. Never hold your breath during a posture. People injure themselves because they move too quickly and forget to breathe. You will find that stretching becomes easier if you move slowly and breathe deeply.

Remind yourself to be patient. Do not be discouraged if you do not seem to be progressing as rapidly as you think you should be. It takes time for the body to become limber. If you are patient and you practice consistently, you will notice a positive difference in the way you feel.

Realize that some parts of your body will be stiffer than others and therefore will need special care and attention. Some people notice that one side of their body tends to be stiffer than the other. Use caution when stretching the stiff side, but always maintain a pose for the same amount of time on each side. If there is any discomfort or pain, either while holding a position or afterward, you are working too hard. Ease up and, again, be patient. Healing is a gradual process.

Journal Entry

I have found that when I feel impatient it is usually because I have in some way "split off" from myself. It means I have placed more importance on an external factor than I have on my peace of mind and self-acceptance.

For me, self-love and self-acceptance are the most important "goals" I can achieve in a day. When I'm feeling impatient with anything I know I'm not loving and accepting myself exactly as I am. I'm looking for an external substitute because I'm not feeling connected and whole.

I appreciate the fact that yoga is such a gentle practice. Nothing is ever forced. It's not a "quick fix", it is a gradual, patient art and it works. I like knowing that gentleness and patience with myself actually get me better results than impatience and force.

Peggy *(Recovering Adult Child)*

Journal Entry

I do yoga in the mornings before I go to work and it makes me feel cleansed and light. It helps me to start off my day with positive thoughts and intentions. With yoga I am much more aware of my breathing patterns. When I am stressed I tend to stop breathing or breathe very shallowly. Now I am conscious of my breath and have been able to transform it into a relaxation tool for stress.

Another thing yoga has helped me with is my self-esteem. I grew up in an alcohol addicted, drug addicted, emotionally abusive environment. Now that I am an adult I find that my self-esteem and confidence are severely low. Yoga has helped me to feel better about myself. As I do yoga I affirm postive thoughts toward my healing. I let go of fear, anger, resentment, and hate. As I stretch and open my body I also open my heart.

Bobbie *(Recovering Adult child)*

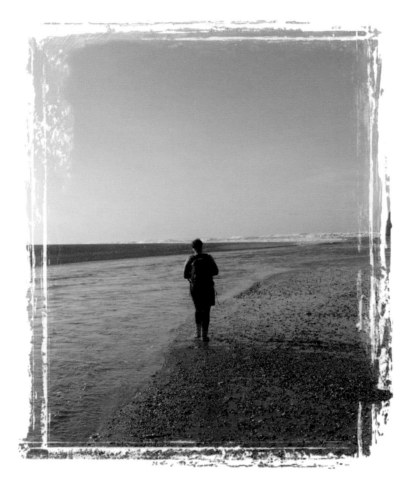

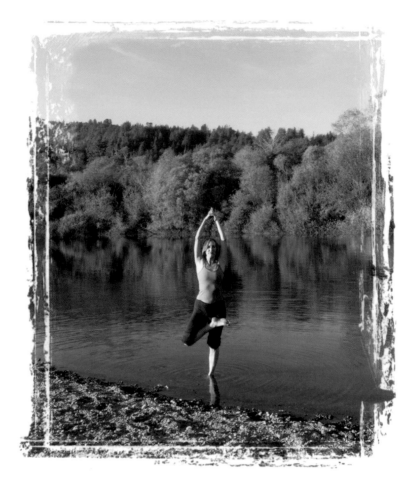

Easy does it.

CHAPTER 4

Yoga Postures with Affirmations

This book is designed for people working a 12-Step program of recovery. The language used refers to the 12 steps. I have not included the Sanskrit names for the postures, and in some cases the pose described is a preparation for the more advanced final pose. For those who wish to investigate yoga and it's advanced forms more fully, there are many excellent books available; several are listed in the Resources at the end of this book. But books are just the place to begin; a teacher is always recommended when you start doing advanced work in yoga. Check your local yellow pages, health clubs, colleges, or YMCAs for leads on local yoga classes. The stretching exercises and postures included here are explained simply and instructively, and offered with encouragement.

Getting Started

For the first month, follow the daily schedule guidelines at the end of this chapter. You will be adding one to three new poses each day, until you have mastered the basics of all 34 poses.

Before you begin, re-read the section on Willingness and Patience at the end of Chapter Three. Then read the directions for doing the poses carefully. Study the photographs and remember that these people have been practicing for some time. Give yourself permission to be a beginner. Move into the postures slowly; find a position you can comfortably hold for a minute or two. Say the affirmation listed beside the pose three times softly or silently to yourself while holding the pose. Remember to breathe deeply and fully, and to coordinate your breathing with your movements. The general rule for breathing is: Breathe in whenever the body expands, opens, or reaches outward; breathe out whenever it contracts, closes, or folds. Breathe through your nose.

Give attentive care to your body and breath as you practice. Do not strain; move gently and comfortably in and out of the poses. If you experience any pain as you do a pose, stop and rest; then consider how you might modify the pose for you. Your breathing will tell you if you are working too hard: if you find you cannot keep a steady deep, full breathing pattern, you need to release your effort a little. All your movements should be slow and deliberate. Come out of each pose slowly. Rest for one or two long deep breaths before moving on to the next pose.

Do not neglect the deep relaxation period that follows the poses. Because it is often easier to relax when listening to instructions, you might want to record one of the relaxation scripts in Chapter Five. You can also use the relaxation CD that I have produced (see ordering instructions at the end of this book). This 30-minute CD includes three visualization-relaxation scripts designed to be played at the end of a yoga class or any time you need 10 minutes of guided relaxation.

And finally, for your comfort, practice Hatha yoga on an empty stomach, at least one-and-a-half hours after your last meal, and wear loose comfortable clothing.

1. STRAIGHT STANDING POSTURE
Standing Mountain

Have you ever noticed that the first impression you get of people is from the way they stand or walk? When people stand straight and walk with their heads high, they appear to be confident, open, and energetic. When people are hunched over, their energy is directed downward and they appear to be unsure of themselves or not as happy as they could be.

One of the first things I realized when I started practicing Hatha yoga is that I had a tendency to hunch my shoulders slightly forward, which made my chest cave in rather than allowing my chest to be open and expanded. It was as if I were subconsciously trying to protect my heart and keep it from being exposed because I had been hurt so often in my life. Changing this habit took a conscious effort on my part, but in time I developed a new stance, which became a symbol of my willingness to face life's challenges with an open heart.

Practice the following straight standing posture often, especially in your daily life when you are standing in lines or standing around with others in conversation.

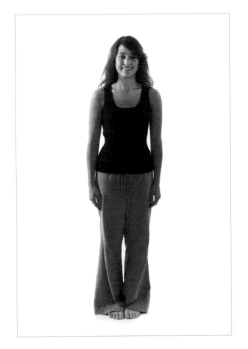

~ I face life's challenges with an open heart ~

INSTRUCTIONS

♦ Begin by standing with your feet parallel.

♦ Rock your weight gently back and forth until you distribute your weight equally through both your feet. Do not lock your knees.

♦ Tuck your tailbone downward toward the floor.

♦ Gently roll your shoulders up and back to lift and separate the rib cage. Then relax your shoulders downward. Let your arms relax by your sides. Your breast bone is lifted up. Your chest is open and relaxed. The back of your neck is light, feeling as though the crown of your head is lifted up toward the sky.

♦ Take several deep breaths.

BENEFITS

Standing Mountain pose increases awareness of body alignment and promotes good standing posture.

2. WARM UP

The Complete Breath with Stretching

INSTRUCTIONS

- Begin in Standing Mountain (straight standing) posture.
- Inhale as you raise your arms above your head, stretching up.
- Exhale bending at the hips, folding forward as you lower your hands down toward the floor in front of you. Let your head hang freely with your neck relaxed. Allow your knees to bend slightly. Exhale all tensions, all worries, all anxiety.
- Inhale and stretch back up, raising your arms above your head, breathing in energy, vitality, and joy.

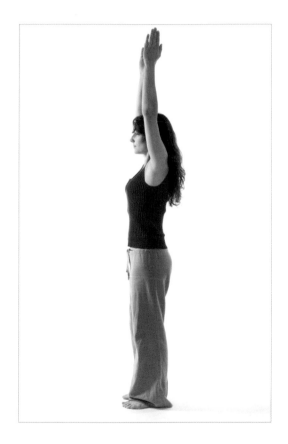

*~ I am filled with energy,
vitality, and joy ~*

- Exhale and fold back down, letting go of all tension, all worries, all doubts.
- Continue breathing in, stretching up; and then breathing out, folding down. Do this five to six times. Focus your thoughts on the affirmations as you do each part.
- With the last exhalation, remain standing while lowering your arms to your sides.

BENEFITS

This Warm Up exercise releases tension in the back and neck and increases energy with breath and movement. It promotes spinal flexibility and stretches the back of the legs.

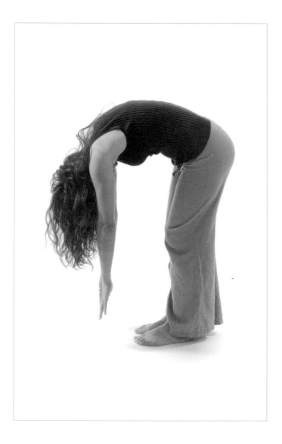

*~ I let go of all tension,
all worries, all anxiety ~*

3. HALF MOON ARCH
Side Stretch

INSTRUCTIONS

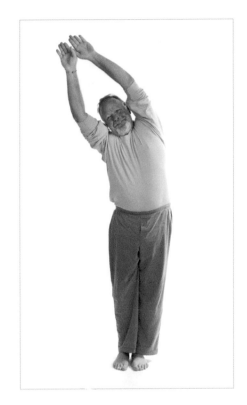

- Stand with your feet parallel and close together, your weight equally distributed on both feet, your arms at your sides.
- Stretch your hands upward, joining them above your head.
- Inhale, lifting up onto your toes as you reach up.
- Exhale, arching over to the left as you lower your heels down. Keep your elbows straight as your arms arch to the left. Do not allow your upper body to twist. The arch extends up and over in alignment with the spine. Keep your weight equally distributed on both feet.
- Hold the pose while breathing and feel the stretch on your right side.

~ Strength and courage flow through me ~

- Inhale up onto your toes as you stretch your hands up above your head.
- Exhale lowering your heels and releasing your arms to your sides.
- Repeat the pose arching to the right, feeling the stretch on your left side.

BENEFITS

This pose strengthens and relaxes the muscles on the sides of your torso. It stretches and tones the muscles along your spine, increasing circulation to the organs. It also strengthens the arches of your feet.

4. ANGLE POSE

INSTRUCTIONS

- Place your feet a little wider than shoulder width apart.
- Turn your left foot out toward the side. Rotate your hips toward your left foot.
- Clasp your hands (interlace fingers) behind your back. Inhale.
- As you exhale, bend at the hips and lower your chest toward your left knee while raising your clasped hands up toward the sky.
- Breathe as you hold the pose.
- Inhale as you rise back up.
- Exhale, releasing your hands and facing forward.
- Repeat the pose on the opposite side.

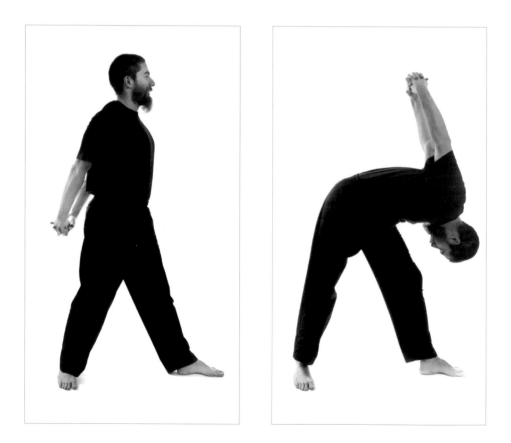

~ I forgive myself and my burdens are lifted ~

- Do the angle stretch a third time, this time facing forward. Place your feet as before.
- Clasp your hands behind your back. Inhale. As you exhale, bend forward while lifting your interlocked arms up toward the sky.
- Exhale lifting back up to standing position and releasing your hands and arms to your sides.

MODIFICATION
- Lift your clasped hands only slightly if you have trouble raising them.

BENEFITS
In this pose, the movements of clasping the hands behind the back, straightening the arms, and lifting them up and away from the body are very beneficial. They rotate the shoulders and help limber the shoulder joints, upper back muscles, and lumbar vertebrae. They also help expand and stretch the rib cage and lungs, which allows fresh blood and energy into the nerves and tissues of the lungs, chest, and heart.

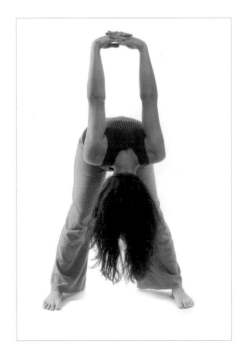

~ I forgive myself and my burdens are lifted ~

5. TRIANGLE POSE

INSTRUCTIONS

Preparing to go into The Triangle

♦ Place your feet shoulder width apart or even a little wider. Turn your left foot out toward the left wall (90 degrees).

♦ Turn your right foot in slightly (30 degrees). The left heel should be in line with the arch of the right foot. Your torso faces forward.

♦ Inhale, raising your arms halfway up, palms down, fingers pointing toward the side walls.

♦ Exhale and shift your pelvis to the right as you reach out to the left, opening the rib cage and extending your torso over your right leg.

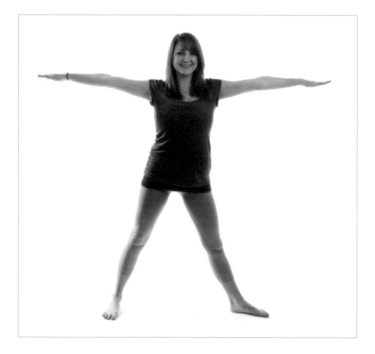

The Triangle

♦ Lower your right hand down to your right thigh or calf while raising your left hand to point toward the sky.

♦ Your left arm is now stretched upward in line with the shoulder, the palm facing forward. Turn your head to look at your left hand as you hold the pose, breathing.

♦ Inhale as you lift back up slowly, facing forward. Turn your feet back to face forward. Exhale as you lower your arms to your sides.
♦ Repeat the pose on the opposite side.

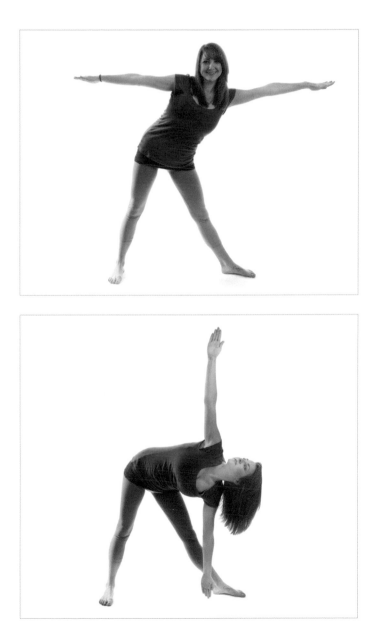

~ I am filled with acceptance and love ~

MODIFICATIONS

◆ If your hamstrings are tight, keep the knee of your leading leg slightly bent while in the pose.

◆ If you have a sensitive neck look forward rather than turning your neck to look at your upper hand while in the pose.

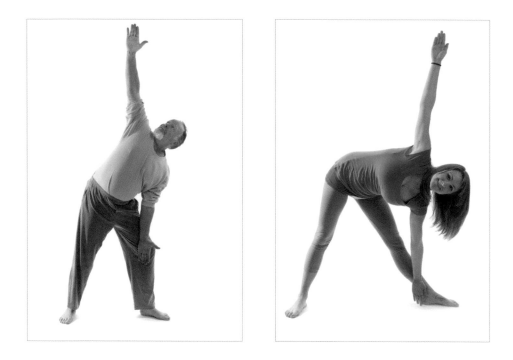

BENEFITS

The Triangle pose stretches the hamstrings and lateral muscles of the spine and stimulates the kidneys and adrenals.

6. THE SQUAT

When I first tried to do the squat it was difficult for me to get my heels flat. I used to wear high heels and my calf muscles were shortened. It took time for me to be able to sit comfortably in this position. People also have problems squatting when their knees are stiff. Yet this pose can be easy and natural. It is a common way to sit in many cultures.

INSTRUCTIONS
Preparing for the Squat
- Place your feet shoulder width apart.
- Bend your knees and reach down. Place your hands on the floor between your feet. Relax your head and neck and breathe.

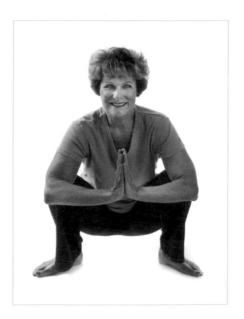

~ I am relaxed and centered ~

The Squat
- Inhale. As you exhale, bend your knees and lower your body down completely into a squat. Your feet should be flat on the floor.
- Bring your palms together in prayer position in front of your chest as you hold the pose, breathing.

Coming out of the Squat

♦ Press your hands on the floor in front of you. Inhale as you straighten
  your legs, raising your buttocks. Exhale as you roll your upper torso
  up slowly, one vertebra at a time.

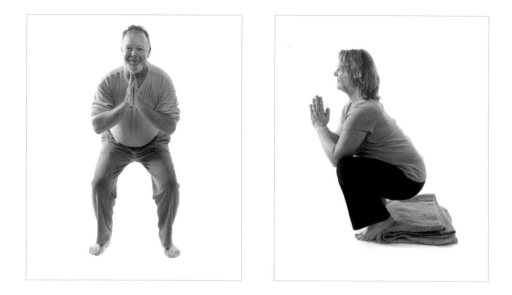

MODIFICATIONS

♦ If you have problems with your knees or hips, proceed cautiously.
  Come halfway down and hold there for several breaths. Go as far as
  you can without straining. Gently work within your limits. You may
  have problems squatting when your knees are stiff. You can do the
  half squat instead.

♦ If you cannot bring your heels flat on the ground, try widening your
  stance. If you are unable to get your heels flat by widening your stance,
  place a rolled-up blanket or yoga mat under your heels for support.

BENEFITS

The squat stretches the calf and thigh muscles and develops balance. It
also helps with digestion and elimination. In the squat, the thighs press
against the colon, which helps to stimulate the bowel function, stimulating the peristaltic movement of materials through the digestive tract.
This pose is especially helpful if you suffer from constipation. It is also
helpful for relieving lower-back discomfort from menstruation.

7. THE WARRIOR

INSTRUCTIONS

- Begin by placing your feet wide apart, as far as is comfortably possible. Your arms should be at your sides.
- Turn your right foot out toward the right wall.
- Turn your left foot in slightly. Inhale, raising your arms up, out to the sides until they are at shoulder level with your palms facing down and your fingers pointing to the side walls.
- Exhale, bending the right knee so that the knee is directly over your ankle, creating a right angle with the floor.
- Keep your torso straight with your spine lifting upward.
- Look toward your right hand while holding the pose and breathing.
- Exhale, releasing your arms, releasing your knee and facing forward.
- Do the pose again on the opposite side.

BENEFITS

Warrior pose gives the feeling of strength and firmness as it tones the arms and legs.

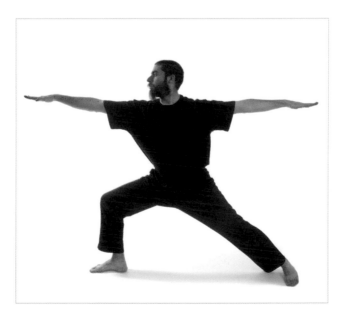

~ I am a warrior of the heart ~

8. THE CHAIR

This is a strengthening pose. It also works with balance. There are two phases to the pose. During both phases, you hold your arms out in front of you. You may get tired of holding them up, but remember that you are strengthening them. This pose strengthens the thighs as well.

INSTRUCTIONS
Phase 1
- Begin with your feet slightly parted, not quite shoulder width apart.
- Extend your arms out in front of you at shoulder level. Inhale.
- As you exhale, bend your knees and sit down as if you are sitting in an imaginary chair.
- Your knees should be directly over your feet, not pointed inward. You are sitting in midair, using your thigh muscles to keep you there. Keep your arms extended forward.
- Remember to breathe as you hold the pose.
- Inhale, straightening your legs.
- Do not drop your arms. Exhale.

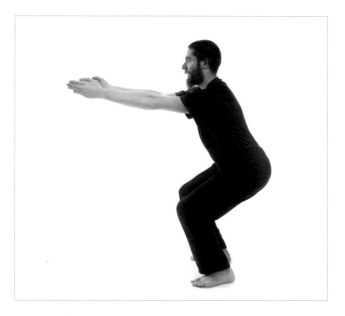

~ My body is the vehicle which houses my soul ~

Phase 2

- Inhale, coming up on your toes. Do not drop your arms.
- As you exhale, sit down again into an imaginary chair, remaining on your toes. Remember to keep your knees directly over your feet. Your arms are still extended forward.
- Breathe. Inhale, straightening your legs to standing position.
- Lower your arms to your sides.

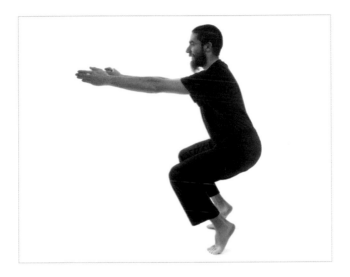

~ My body is the vehicle which houses my soul ~

CAUTION

Do not overdo this. If you have "problem knees" or find this pose too difficult you can skip this position or do the modification below. As you develop strength in your leg muscles it will become easier to do.

MODIFICATION

- If you have knee problems then remain standing and do the arm part of the posture only, while focusing your thoughts on the affirmation.

BENEFITS

Chair pose strengthens and tones the arms and legs. It also helps improve balance.

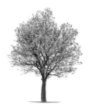

9. THE TREE

This is a balancing pose. When you think about trees, they are wonderful examples of balance. A tree has deep roots in the earth, a strong sturdy trunk, and branches that are very expansive and lift up toward the sky. When storms come the tree bends with the wind. In fact, branches that are not flexible, but are stiff and rigid, often break in the storm. We human beings are the same way. When the storms of stress hit our lives we need to remain rooted in who we are, in our divine nature and what that means to us; yet we also need to be flexible with the changes that life brings to us, for if we remain rigid and tense with resistance we too will break and fall.

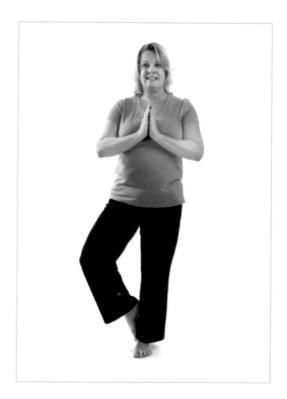

INSTRUCTIONS

♦ Begin by placing your weight on your left foot. Visualize roots growing from the bottom of your left foot going deep into the earth. Focus on a stationary point in front of you.

♦ Place your right foot on your left calf or thigh. Inhale and place your hands in prayer position at your heart or raise them up above your head, reaching for the sky.

♦ Exhale, releasing your arms and your foot. Repeat the pose on the opposite foot.

BENEFITS

The Tree helps develop concentration, balance, and poise.

NOTE

Don't feel bad if you have a difficult time keeping your balance in the beginning. Work with it. Try using a plant or tree as your point of focus. In time your balance will improve.

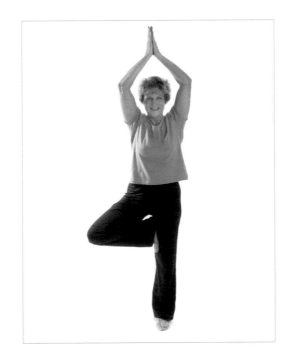

~ I am calm, I am balanced, I am rooted in faith ~

10. THE SITTING MOUNTAIN

This is one of the easiest ways to sit so that your spine remains straight rather than hunched over.

INSTRUCTIONS
- Kneel on the floor and sit back on your heels. Your toes should be touching and your heels separated.
- Keep your back upright. Relax your shoulders.
- Chest is open and relaxed. You are firmly planted like a mountain, energy going up your spine, feeling strong and calm.
- Take deep slow breaths.

MODIFICATIONS
- If your thighs are tight and sitting on your feet is painful, place a pillow or folded blanket between your buttocks and your heels. If you have knee problems, you can do this pose sitting in a chair, keeping your chest open and relaxed with spine straight.

BENEFITS
This is a meditative pose that flushes blood from the legs as it stretches the hips, knees and ankle joints.

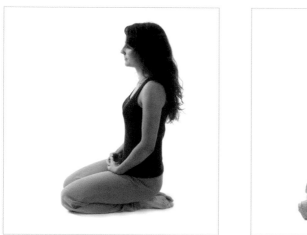
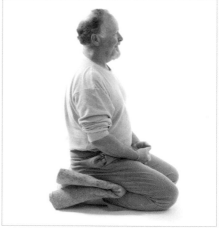

~ Serenity comes when I surrender ~

11. CHILD'S POSE

INSTRUCTIONS

◆ Begin in Sitting Mountain pose, kneeling with thighs on calves, sitting on your feet with your toes touching and your heels separated. Inhale.

◆ As you exhale, gently lower your head to the floor in front of your knees.

◆ Forehead rests on the floor. Place your hands, palms up, next to your feet.

◆ Completely relax your neck and shoulders. Hold this position while breathing for as long as you are comfortable.

◆ Inhale, coming back to Sitting Mountain pose.

BENEFITS

Child's pose allows the blood to flow to the neck and head. This pose releases tension in the shoulders and spine. It gently allows blood flow to the brain, relieving mental fatigue.

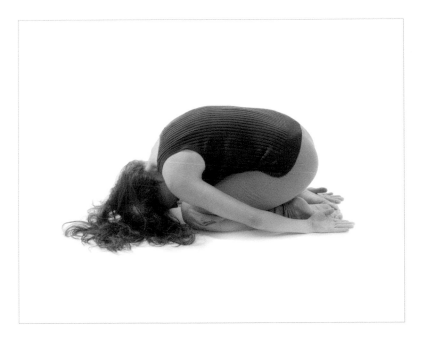

~ I rest in trust and patience ~

12. THE COBRA

INSTRUCTIONS

Preparing to go into the cobra

♦ Lie on your stomach, with your forehead on the floor. Your body should be fully extended with your legs and feet together, toes pointed.

♦ Place your palms on the floor directly underneath your shoulders, fingers pointed forward. Keep your arms close to your rib cage and your elbows pointing upward.

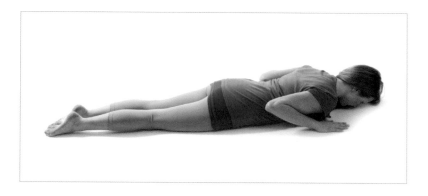

Phase one

♦ Inhale and raise your head slowly upward. Raise your chest slightly off the floor without putting pressure on your hands. Use your upper back to hold the pose. Your hands are used for support only. Hold here for five seconds, breathing.

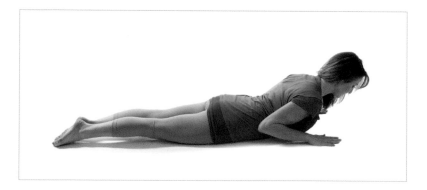

Phase two: full cobra

♦ Now gently push against the floor with your palms, tighten the muscles in your legs and buttocks, and slowly lift your chest to create a backward arch.

♦ Keep your elbows bent in close to your body and your pelvis on the floor. Relax your shoulders and hold the pose while breathing.

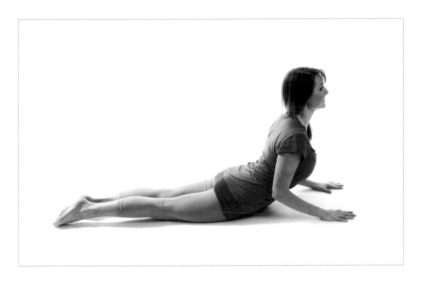

~ I calmly rise to greet each moment ~

♦ Exhale and slowly lower your chest and forehead to the floor.
♦ Turn your cheek to the side.
♦ Place your arms down along side your body and rest.

BENEFITS

The Cobra strengthens the upper back and vertebrae of the spine. It expands the rib cage and increases the capacity of the lungs.

13. LYING DOWN BOAT

INSTRUCTIONS

- Lie on your stomach with your chin on the floor. Extend your arms forward, resting them on the floor. Your feet and legs should be close together and relaxed.
- Inhaling, raise your arms and legs off the floor, arching up until only your stomach remains on the floor.
- Tighten your buttocks and hold the pose, just for a moment at first, and gradually over time for up to three breaths.
- Exhale, lower your body, and relax.

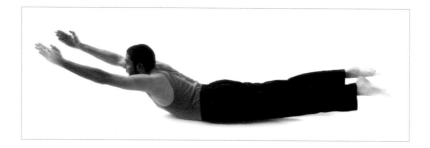

~ I reach out to others when I need help ~

MODIFICATION

- If it is difficult for you to extend your arms forward you can do the pose with your arms along side your back, lifting up.

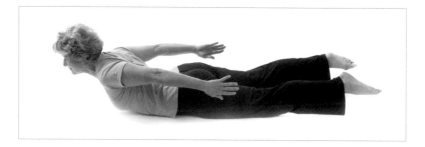

BENEFITS

This pose helps to strengthen the lower back.

14. THE CAT

INSTRUCTIONS

♦ This pose alternates between swayback and humpback. Kneel on all fours with your arms straight and your back parallel to the floor. As you inhale, lift your head and tailbone up, and allow your waist to lower into swayback.

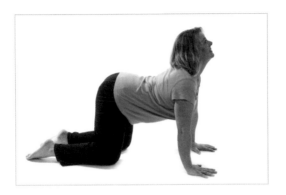

~ I have the option to change my attitude ~

♦ Hold this position for three seconds.
♦ As you exhale, hunch and round your back, lower your tailbone and let your head relax down. Hold this position for three seconds.

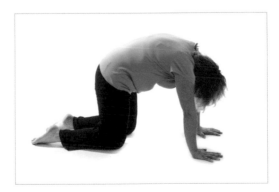

BENEFITS

The Cat helps stretch and strengthen the spine.

15. BACKWARD BEND

INSTRUCTIONS

♦ Start in Sitting Mountain pose, sitting on your heels, with the tops of your feet resting on the floor and your knees together in front of you.

♦ Relax your shoulders and lift your chest. Place your hands beside you, palms face down, fingers pointed back.

♦ Little by little, walk your hands back until you reach a comfortable position where you are leaning back on your arms.

♦ Relax your head and neck as you lift your chest and ribs toward the ceiling to create an arch. Remain seated on your heels and breathe as you hold the pose.

♦ Release the pose by slowly shifting your chest and ribs forward, while raising your head until your chin touches your chest. Walk your hands forward to a sitting position.

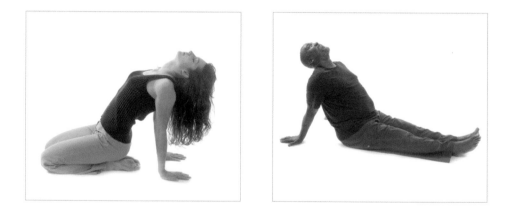

~ I lean on God for guidance ~

MODIFICATION

♦ If it is difficult for you to kneel you can do this pose with your legs extended out in front of you.

BENEFITS

Backward Bend promotes elasticity in the spine. It stretches and lengthens the muscles across the chest. It also tones the neck and throat.

16. THE CAMEL (PREPARATION)

INSTRUCTIONS

- Kneel, sitting on your heels with your spine straight.
- Inhale and rise upward so that you are still on your knees, with your body erect over your knees. Separate your knees slightly.
- Place your hands on your lower back and arch your spine, lifting your sternum and expanding your chest.
- Slowly release your hands and lift back up to an erect kneeling position. Lower your body. Fold forward into the Child's Pose.

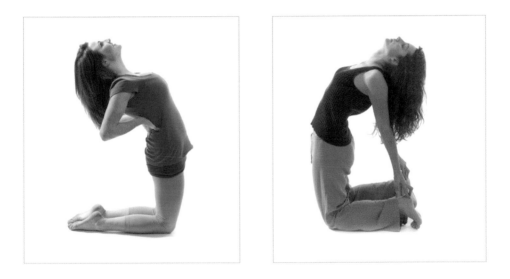

~ I am open and receptive to life's lessons ~

MODIFICATION (ADVANCED)

- You can begin to move further into camel pose by curling your toes so that your heals are up and within reach of your hands. Bend back to touch the heals while keeping your thighs forward. Lift the sternum and let the head relax back.

BENEFITS

The Camel Preparation pose expands the chest and stretches the shoulders. It is helpful for people who tend to round their shoulders.

17. DOWNWARD FACING DOG

INSTRUCTIONS

♦ Begin in The Table pose, on all fours. Spread your fingers wide apart and keep your hands pressed against the floor beneath your shoulders. Your arms are straight. Your back is parallel to the floor.

♦ Tuck your toes under. Inhale.

♦ As you exhale press your palms against the floor as you straighten your legs, lifting your buttocks toward the ceiling. Stay high on your toes and press your chest toward your thighs.

♦ Your abdomen lifts up as you push your weight back into your legs, extending your spine.

♦ Slowly lower your heels toward the floor.

♦ Keep pressing your palms into the floor. Drop your head down. Relax your shoulders away from your neck. Breathe.

♦ Release your knees to the floor; then sit up.

BENEFITS

This pose gives an intense stretch to the back of the legs, especially the calves.

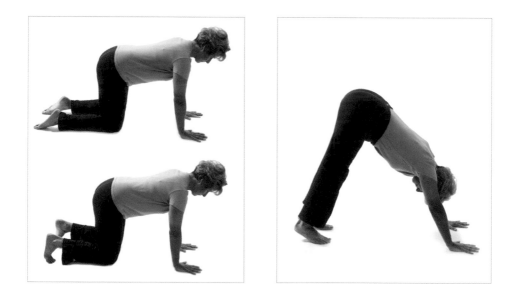

~ I have faith in the unknown before me ~

18. HEAD TO KNEE POSE

INSTRUCTIONS

♦ Sit up straight on the floor with your legs extended out in front of you.

♦ Bend your right knee and place the sole of your right foot against your left inner thigh. Flex your left foot.

♦ Inhale, raising your arms up above your head.

♦ Exhale, bending at your hips, lowering your chest and head toward your left knee.

♦ Bring your hands down to your left calf, ankle, or foot, wherever you can comfortably reach.

♦ Hold the pose while breathing.

♦ Inhale, lifting your arms up above your head as you come out of the pose.

♦ Exhale, releasing your arms to your sides.

♦ Repeat the pose with your right leg extended and your left knee bent.

BENEFITS

The Head to Knee pose stretches the hamstrings, knees, and lower back.

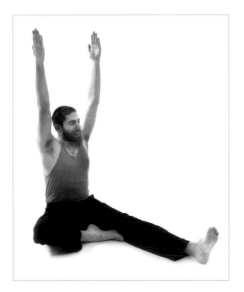 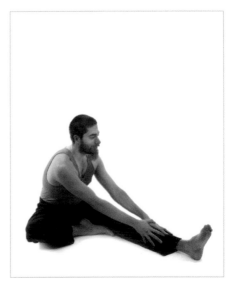

~ Everything I need I possess in this moment ~

19. SEATED FORWARD BEND

INSTRUCTIONS

♦ Sit on the floor with your legs extended out in front of you. Rotate your
ankles, flexing and stretching them to loosen them up. Sit up straight
and flex your feet. Inhale, raising your arms up above your head.

♦ Exhale, bending at the hips, lowering your chest toward your knees.
Keep your spine straight as you do this. Place your hands on your
knees, calves, ankles, or feet, wherever you can comfortably reach.

♦ Keep your feet flexed. Hold the pose while breathing.

♦ Inhale, raising your arms straight up above your head as you sit up.

♦ Exhale, lowering your arms to your sides.

MODIFICATION

♦ Place a strap around the balls of your feet to help keep your spine
straight while stretching in this pose.

BENEFITS

This pose helps limber the hamstrings and lower back.

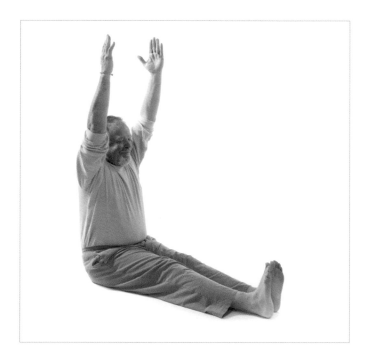

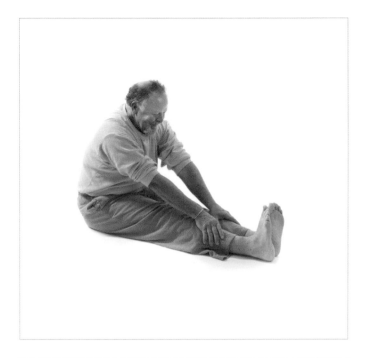

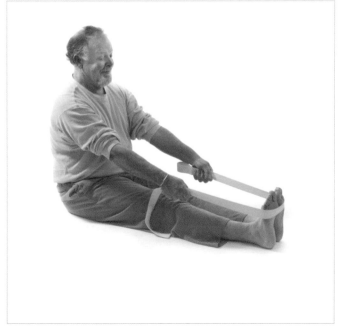

~ I move forward with patience ~

20. THE BUTTERFLY

INSTRUCTIONS

♦ Sit up straight. Place the bottoms of your feet together, pulling them in toward your groin. Your knees should be out to your sides.

♦ Inhale. As you exhale, lean forward.

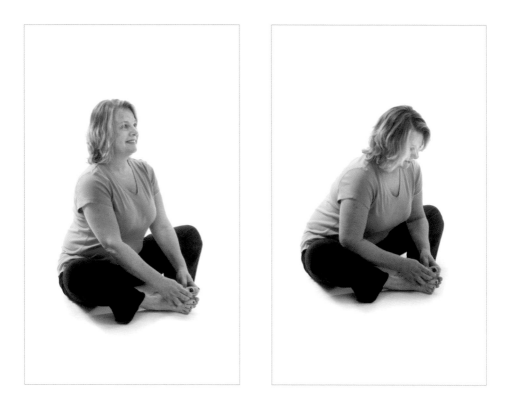

~ My spirit is as gentle as a butterfly ~

♦ Clasp your feet and begin pressing your forearms into your calves and knees, gently pushing your knees toward the floor.

♦ Hold the pose while continuing to press your knees down. Breathe.

♦ Inhale, sitting back up and releasing your knees

BENEFITS

The Butterfly pose works to gently open the pelvis.

21. INNER THIGH STRETCH
V Position

INSTRUCTIONS

- Sit on the floor with your legs extended out in front of you. Spread your legs out into a V position, as wide as is comfortable. Flex your feet (bend your knees slightly if you like).
- Inhale, sitting up straight.
- Exhale and lean forward as you slowly walk your hands out away from you. You are attempting to lower your chest toward the floor. Breathe.
- After several breaths, walk your hands back up and slide your legs together in front of you.

BENEFITS

Inner Thigh Stretch improves inner-thigh flexibility and loosens the hip joints.

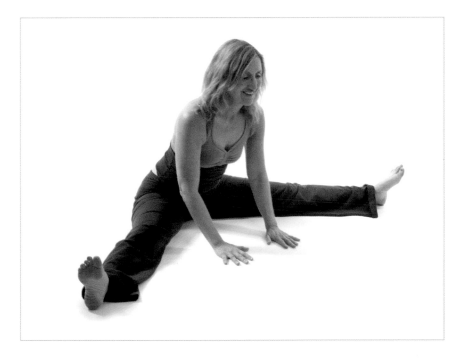

~ Nonresistance gives me peace ~

22. ROCK THE BABY

INSTRUCTIONS

♦ Sit up straight on the floor with your legs extended forward.
♦ Raise your right leg and bend it toward you.
♦ Place both arms around your leg as if you were cradling a baby, your right foot is in the bend of your left elbow and your knee is in the bend of your right elbow.

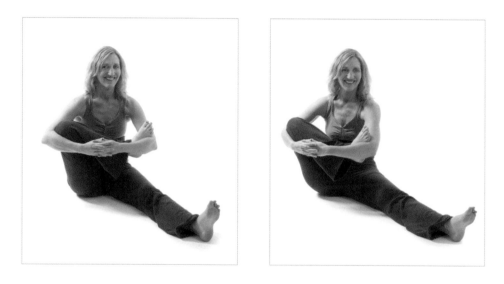

~ I gently open to my inner wisdom ~

♦ If you can reach easily, interlace your fingers.
♦ Gently rock your leg from side to side.
♦ Release your leg and sit with your legs extended. Repeat on the other side.

BENEFITS

Rock the Baby loosens the hip joint, opens the groin, and stretches the outer thigh.

23. GENTLE SPINAL TWIST

INSTRUCTIONS

♦ Sit on the floor with your legs crossed. Place your left hand on your right knee. Extend your right arm out to the side. Inhale.

♦ As you exhale, twist to the right bringing your right arm around behind your back and resting your right hand on your left inner thigh, if you can reach that far.

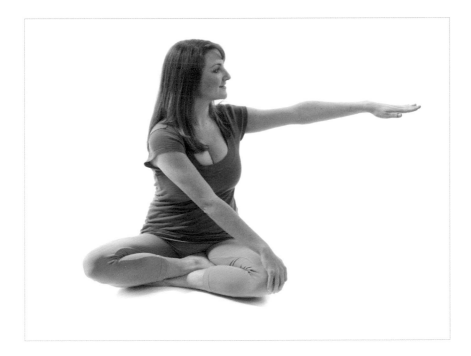

~ I let go of the past with forgiveness ~

♦ Look over your right shoulder. Breathe.
♦ Exhale, releasing the pose.
♦ Repeat the pose, twisting to the left.

BENEFITS

Gentle Spinal Twist increases elasticity of the spine.

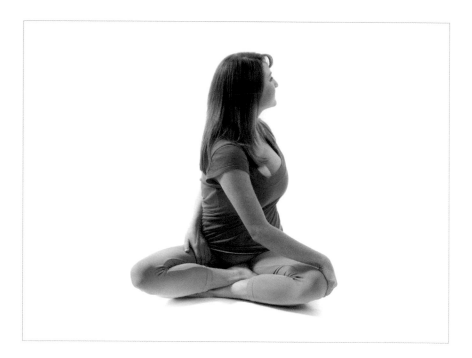

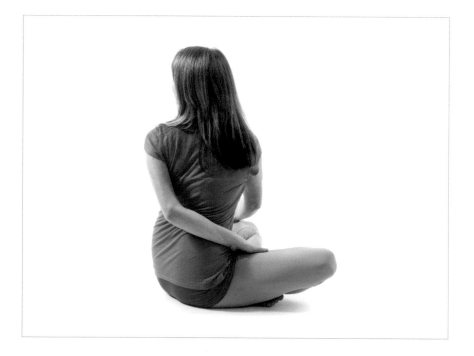

~ I let go of the past with forgiveness ~

24. SITTING BOAT

INSTRUCTIONS

- Lie on your back with your legs together and your arms beside your body. Take a deep breath.
- As you exhale, raise both legs and your upper body until you are balancing on your hips.
- Extend your arms forward, parallel to the floor, reaching toward your toes.
- Hold the pose for just a moment at first, then gradually work up to holding it for several breaths.
- Release, lie down, and relax.

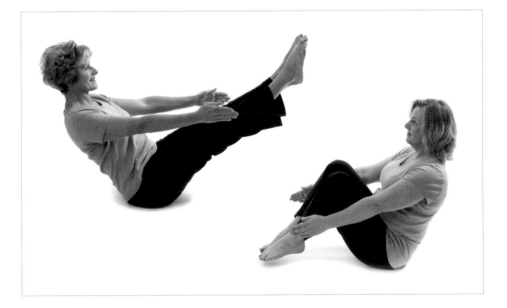

~ My Higher Power gives me inner strength ~

MODIFICATION

- If you have strain in your lower back, then keep your knees bent in the pose.

BENEFITS

Sitting Boat pose helps to strengthen the stomach muscles.

25. LITTLE BOAT (HUGGING KNEES)

INSTRUCTIONS
- Lie on your back. Bring your knees in toward your chest.
- Wrap your arms around your knees and legs, hugging them in toward your chest.
- Keep your chin slightly tucked so your neck is lengthened. Hold the position and breathe.
- Release you legs and arms so that you are lying down on your back.

BENEFITS
Little Boat pose releases the lower back and lengthens the spine.

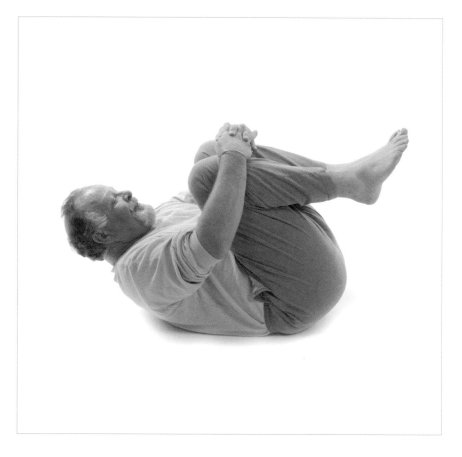

~ I trust myself ~

26. GENTLE PELVIC ROCKING

INSTRUCTIONS

- Lie on your back. Bend your knees, placing your feet flat on the floor hip width apart. Draw them in toward your buttocks so that your knees are pointed upward, side by side.
- Inhale, pressing your lower back into the floor. Tighten your buttocks and roll one or two of your lowest vertebrae off the floor, just lifting your tailbone slightly. You are curling your pelvis toward the ceiling while pressing your back into the floor.
- Exhale, pressing your tailbone back down toward the floor so that your lower back arches.
- Inhale, pressing your lower back in the floor, tightening your buttocks, and lifting your tailbone slightly again.
- Exhale, releasing your tailbone allowing your lower back to arch. Continue rocking your pelvis gently and slowly 9 to 10 times.

BENEFITS

Gentle Pelvic Rocking increases the strength and suppleness of the pelvic region while toning the buttocks.

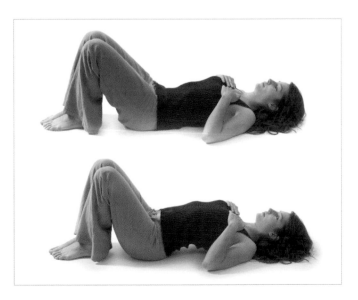

~ I like myself unconditionally ~

27. SLANT BOARD

INSTRUCTIONS

♦ Lie on your back and place your feet flat on the floor, drawing them in toward your buttocks so that your knees are pointed upward.

♦ Inhale, and press your lower back into the floor.

♦ Exhale, lifting your tailbone and lifting your vertebrae slowly, your thighs lifting up so that you create a slant, a straight line from your knees to your shoulders.

♦ Your chin is tucked into your chest. Hold the pose while breathing.

♦ Exhale, coming back down slowly, one vertebra at a time, beginning with your upper back and ending with your lower back, pressing into the floor.

BENEFITS

Slant Board pose stretches the spine and releases neck tension. It reverses the pull of gravity, allowing blood to flow toward the chest, neck, and head.

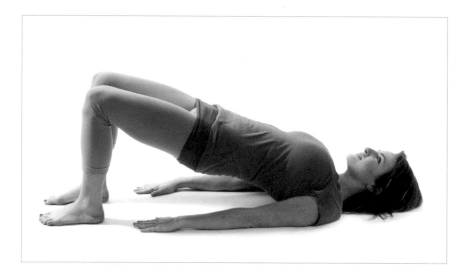

~ Honesty is my commitment to myself ~

28. THE ARCH

INSTRUCTIONS

- Lie on your back with your knees bent and your feet flat on the floor. Place your feet hip-width apart, drawing them in toward your buttocks with your knees pointed upward.
- Inhale, pressing your lower back into the floor.
- Exhale, lift your tailbone and continue lifting your spine up into an arch. Press your feet into the floor, lifting your thighs and stomach up high. Clasp your hands underneath your back, and interlace your fingers. Straighten your arms.
- Your chin is tucked. Hold the pose while breathing.
- Exhale, releasing your hands and coming down one vertebra at a time from the top of your shoulders all the way down to your tailbone.
- Take a deep breath and release it. Pull your knees into your chest for a moment. Then extend your legs and relax.

BENEFITS

The Arch increases flexibility in the spine and shoulders and develops strength in the lower back and stomach. It also releases tension in the abdomen.

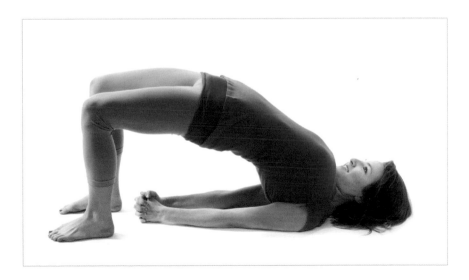

~ I am uplifted as I live in truth ~

29. KNEE HUG SPINAL TWIST

INSTRUCTIONS

♦ Lie on your back and hug your knees into your chest. Keep your knees bent into your chest, and place your arms out to your sides, (palms can be faced up or down), Inhale.

♦ Exhale, twisting your knees to the right as you turn your head to the left. Hold the position and breathe.

♦ Inhale, moving your knees and head back to the center.

♦ Exhale, twisting your knees to the left and your head to the right.

♦ Hold the position and breathe.

♦ Inhale, moving your knees and head back to the center. Release your legs and lie flat. Relax.

BENEFITS

This pose stretches and tones the spinal ligaments, releasing energy in the spine and increasing flexibility of the spine, back, and ribs.

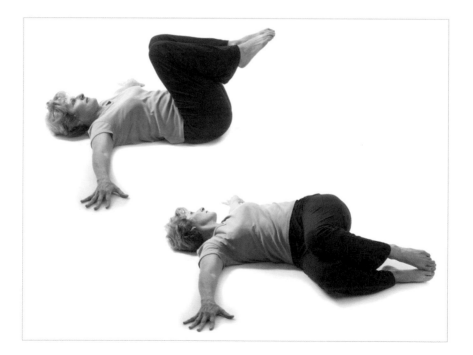

~ Everywhere I turn I see beauty ~

30. HALF PLOUGH

INSTRUCTIONS

- Lie on your back, placing your arms along the sides of your body with your palms facing down and your legs together.
- Bring your knees up to your abdomen. Then, straighten them toward the ceiling.
- Exhale, pushing against the floor with your hands as you lift your torso.
- Raise your hips off the floor and extend your feet behind your head until your legs are parallel to the floor. Support your lower back with your hands.
- Your chin should be tucked into your chest. Breathe evenly as you hold the pose.

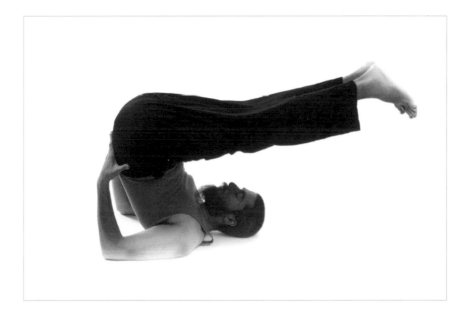

~ I am grateful for this moment of life ~

- Exhale and slowly lower your hips. Return your legs to perpendicular position.
- Continue exhaling as you slowly lower your legs to the floor.

MODIFICATION

♦ For increased support of your neck, place a folded blanket on the floor and lie on your back with the top of your shoulders below the folded edge of the blanket. Position yourself so that the back of your neck does not touch the floor. If necessary add another folded blanket. Then go into the pose.

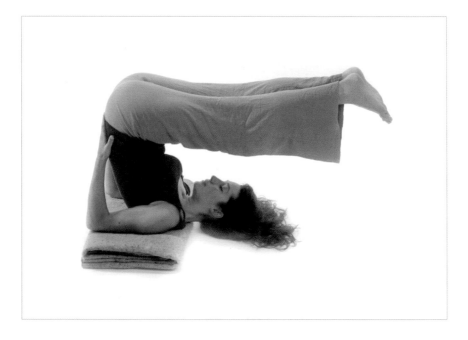

BENEFITS

Half Plough pose promotes spinal flexibility and deep relaxation of all the muscles. It improves the functioning of the internal organs by supplying them with extra blood.

CAUTION

Do not attempt the half plough if you have high blood pressure, have a sinus infection, have a loose retina, are menstruating, or have a weak or injured neck or lower back.

31. SIMPLE INVERTED POSE

INSTRUCTIONS

♦ Lie on your back. Inhale and slowly raise your legs up so that they are perpendicular to the floor.

♦ Keeping your legs in a vertical position, slowly raise your hips until you can support them with your hands.

♦ Keep your thumbs on your sides and place your elbows on the floor about a foot apart; if your elbows are too far apart, they will not give adequate support to your body, which is resting on them.

♦ Your neck is free. The weight of the pose should be on your elbows, not your neck. Keep your legs straight and toes pointed. Hold the pose while breathing.

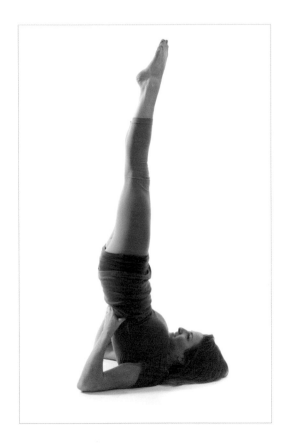

~ I accept all of my feelings as a part of myself ~

♦ Exhale, slowly lowering your hips and returning your legs to a perpendicular position. Continue exhaling and slowly lower your legs to the floor.

MODIFICATION

♦ If you are unable to do Simple Inverted Pose, substitute Leg Inversion against the Wall (see next exercise).

BENEFITS

Simple Inverted Pose helps reverse the pull of gravity. It relaxes the legs by relieving pressure. It allows blood to flow into the upper body, giving the glands and organs a lift.

CAUTION

Do not attempt the inverted pose if you have high blood pressure, have ear, eye, or nose infections, glaucoma, a loose retina, brain injury, or are menstruating.

32. LEG INVERSION AGAINST THE WALL

If you are unable to do the Simple Inverted Pose, this is a great substitute.

INSTRUCTIONS

♦ Lie on the floor beside an empty wall, with your knees bent and your left hip touching the wall so that your side is against the wall.

♦ Slide your legs up the wall as you turn your body toward the wall.

♦ Keep your buttocks against the wall and lie with your torso on the floor and your legs elevated against the wall.

♦ Straighten your legs.

♦ Hold the pose and breathe.

♦ Bend your knees and lower your legs beside the wall.

♦ Move away from the wall and lie down on your back.

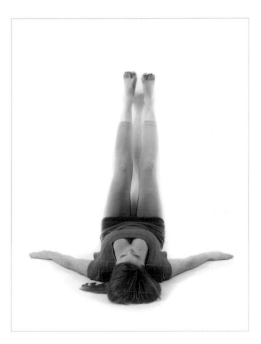

~ As I relax, I gain insight, clarity, and ease ~

MODIFICATION

♦ Place a pillow under your head and buttocks for more support.

BENEFITS

Leg Inversion Against The Wall relaxes the legs and feet by relieving pressure.

33. FISH

This pose is a counter pose to the *Simple Inverted Pose (31)* and *Half Plough (30)*, bending your neck and head in the opposite direction. You need strong back muscles to hold the lift of your upper back in the arched Fish pose.

INSTRUCTIONS
- Lie on your back. Place your hands under your buttocks, palms up, and inhale.
- Exhale as you press your elbows and forearms into the floor and lift your sternum or breastbone away from the floor.
- Arch your back. Stretch your neck backward, resting the crown of your head on the floor. Hold the pose while breathing evenly.
- Slowly lower your shoulders and neck to the ground. Relax.

MODIFICATION
- If you are a beginner, have back pain, or have a weak upper back, substitute *The Camel (Preparation) Pose (16)*.

BENEFITS
Fish pose relieves a stiff neck, opens the breathing cavity, opens the shoulders, and relieves tension in the throat.

CAUTION
If your neck hurts, lower your shoulders and neck to the ground and release the pose. Do not push yourself beyond your limits.

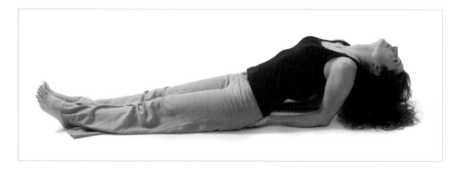

~ I breathe easily as I release control ~

34. CORPSE POSE

INSTRUCTIONS

♦ Lie on your back and gently close your eyes.
♦ Place your feet and legs slightly apart.
♦ Place your arms along the sides of your body with your palms facing up. Make sure your teeth are slightly parted so that your jaw is relaxed.
♦ Start taking some deep breaths. In the pose your body should resemble a corpse, lying still and relaxed.
♦ Stay in this position for 5 to 10 minutes.

BENEFITS

Corpse Pose is the basic pose of relaxation that is done at the end of each Hatha yoga session. It helps relieve the body of tension, and it relieves the body and mind of fatigue. It relaxes, rejuvenates, and replenishes the mind and body.

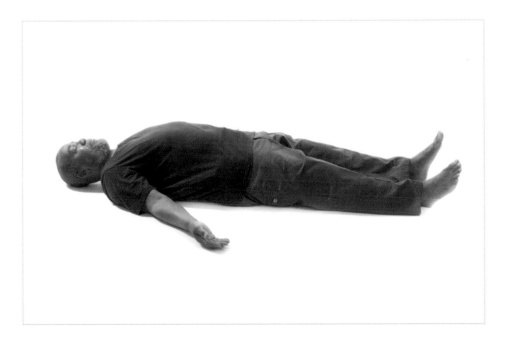

~ I allow myself to relax completely,
I surrender to my Higher Power ~

Four-Week Suggested Routine
Week One

DAY 1
- Straight standing posture
- Warm up
- Half moon arch
- Angle stretch
- Corpse

DAY 2
- Straight standing posture
- Warm up
- Half moon arch
- Angle stretch
- Triangle
- Corpse

DAY 3
- Straight standing posture
- Warm up
- Half moon arch
- Angle stretch
- Triangle
- Squat
- Corpse

DAY 4
- Warm up
- Half moon arch
- Angle stretch
- Triangle
- Squat
- Warrior
- Corpse

DAY 5
- Warm up
- Half moon arch
- Angle stretch
- Warrior
- Chair
- Tree
- Corpse

DAY 6
- Warm up
- Half moon arch
- Triangle
- Warrior
- Chair
- Tree
- Corpse

DAY 7
- Rest

Four-Week Suggested Routine
Week Two

DAY 8
- Warm up
- Tree
- Sitting mountain
- Child's pose
- Cobra
- Cat
- Corpse

DAY 9
- Warm Up
- Half moon arch
- Angle Pose
- Sitting mountain
- Cobra
- Backward bend
- Child's pose
- Corpse

DAY 10
- Warm up
- Sitting mountain
- Cobra
- Lying down boat
- Cat
- Backward bend
- Child's pose
- Downward dog
- Corpse

DAY 11
- Warm up
- Sitting mountain
- Child's pose
- Cobra
- Lying boat
- Cat
- Head to knee
- Seated forward bend
- Corpse

DAY 12
- Warm up
- Child's pose
- Cat
- Backward bend
- Camel preparation
- Downward dog
- Head to knee
- Seated forward bend
- Corpse

DAY 13
- Warm up
- Child's pose
- Cobra
- Lying boat
- Cat
- Backward bend
- Camel preparation
- Downward dog
- Head to knee
- Seated forward bend
- Corpse

DAY 14
- Rest

Four-Week Suggested Routine
Week Three

DAY 15
- Warm up
- Head to knee
- Sitting forward Bend
- Butterfly
- Inner thigh stretch
- Rock the baby
- Gentle spinal twist
- Corpse

DAY 16
- Warm up
- Seated forward bend
- Butterfly
- Inner thigh stretch
- Rock the baby
- Sitting boat
- Little boat
- Knee hugging spinal twist
- Corpse

DAY 17
- Warm up
- Head to knee
- Seated forward bend
- Butterfly
- Inner thigh
- Rock the baby
- Gentle spinal twist
- Sitting boat
- Gentle pelvic rocking
- Corpse

DAY 18
- Warm up
- Half moon arch
- Chair
- Tree
- Seated forward bend
- Butterfly
- Inner thigh
- Gentle pelvic rocking
- Slant board
- Knee hug spinal twist
- Corpse

DAY 19
- Warm up
- Downward dog
- Child's pose
- Head to knee
- Seated forward bend
- Gentle pelvic rocking
- Slant board
- Arch
- Knee hug spinal twist
- Leg inversion agaist wall
- Corpse

DAY 20
- Warm up
- Inner thigh stretch
- Rock the baby
- Gentle spinal twist
- Sitting boat
- Gentle pelvic rocking
- Slant board
- Arch
- Half plough
- Leg inversion against wall
- Corpse

DAY 21
- Rest

Four-Week Suggested Routine
Week Four

DAY 22
- Warm up
- Half moon arch
- Angle stretch
- Triangle
- Squat
- Warrior
- Sitting mountain
- Child's pose
- Corpse

DAY 23
- Downward dog
- Sitting mountain
- Backward bend
- Camel preparation
- Child's pose
- Cobra
- Lying down boat
- Cat
- Corpse

DAY 24
- Mountain
- Child's Pose
- Cobra
- Lying down boat
- Sitting boat
- Little boat
- Gentle pelvic rocking
- Slant
- Arch
- Knee hugging spinal twist
- Corpse

DAY 25
- Warm up
- Side stretch
- Angle stretch
- Triangle

- Chair
- Tree
- Seated forward bend
- Half plough
- Simple inverted pose
- Fish
- Corpse

DAY 26
- Warm up
- Half moon arch
- Triangle
- Tree
- Cat
- Backward bend
- Camel
- Downward dog
- Child's pose
- Leg Inversion against wall
- Corpse

DAY 27
- Warm up
- Cat
- Downward dog
- Seated forward bend
- Butterfly
- Inner thigh stretch
- Sitting boat
- Lying boat
- Cobra
- Child's Pose
- Knee hugging spinal twist
- Half plough
- Simple inverted pose
- Fish
- Corpse

DAY 2
- Rest

Weeks Five and Onward

You are now familiar with all of the yoga postures. Continue following the suggested four week routine until you are comfortable with all the postures. After a while, your body will tell you which posture it needs or wants to do, and you will start to develop your own routine. In other words, you will begin to sense which areas in your body need stretching, strengthening, and opening. You will know which postures would be the most beneficial for you at any given time. Do bear in mind, though, that the body is inherently lazy — it prefers to do things that are easy. So when you develop your routine, don't neglect groups of poses because they are not your favorites. Balance and wholeness are your goals, so include some back bending as well as some forward bending, some standing poses as well as sitting poses, and so on.

Keep in mind that Hatha yoga teaches care and appreciation of the body. When you practice the postures your body becomes strong and flexible, and you have more energy. If you stop the routine you will notice the difference: more stiffness, less energy, less flexibility. When this happens realize that all it takes is one day of stretching to remember how good it feels and motivate you back into your routine. Think of the postures as an important part of your recovery that are helping your body to heal from stress; approach the practice one day at a time. Allow simply 10 to 20 minutes of stretching followed with relaxation each day and you will be rewarded with greater ease and well being.

Always begin your practice with the breathing and stretching warm up exercises instructed on page 53. Remember that the breath is a key ingredient to Hatha yoga. Deep, full breathing prepares the body for the yoga postures by warming and relaxing the muscles. Regardless of which posture you are practicing, the breath will aid you in releasing tension and will help promote the stretching and opening of the body.

When you are finished with your daily session of postures, allow at least five minutes for complete relaxation. Chapter five describes specific techniques. When time permits, follow relaxation with prayer, meditation, and journal writing. These practices will shift your self-awareness toward humility and peace.

Journal Entry

Yoga helps me in my recovery because it gives balance to my life. I am a compulsive workaholic. Workaholism is no different than any other addiction. It affects my relationships, it saps my physical well being, it provides an alluring, but false, sense of self-esteem.

Practicing yoga poses takes the edge off the compulsion that surrounds my addiction. Usually my mind is going ten directions at once, but when I practice yoga I stop worrying about all the things I have to do, and I allow myself to just "be." I bring my attention to my body and my breath. I notice where my body feels stiff and tight. I seem to carry lots of tension in my neck and shoulders.

As I begin to stretch I release the tension in my body. I stop thinking so much, staying in my head and intellect; and I move into feeling my body and emotions. I can actually feel my muscles relax as I stretch and breathe.

I like the affirmations as well, because they also help to calm my mind. Sometimes when I am working, I stop amidst all the compulsion to push harder and accomplish more, and just breathe deep from my lower abdomen. Often my favorite yoga affirmation "honesty is my commitment to myself" will accompany my breath. I inhale honesty and exhale fear, reminding myself to slow down and relax.

Sam *(Workaholic)*

Journal Entry

Tonight I came to yoga class with so much pain and tension. My back and neck were in spasms and I had been experiencing migraine headaches all day. I had such a hard time accepting my pain. I wanted to get my prescription drugs to kill the pain, but I can't do that anymore. Sometimes I feel like screaming, "Life is unfair!"

Thank God for yoga. When I stretch my body and say the affirmations I become more forgiving to myself and my body. The deep breathing really helps with the pain so it doesn't seem so unbearable. As I begin to relax I can feel the release of discomfort. It's amazing. I've got to remember to use the yoga techniques. Yoga is so much healthier than my desire to ingest pain killers.

Mary *(Recovering Addict)*

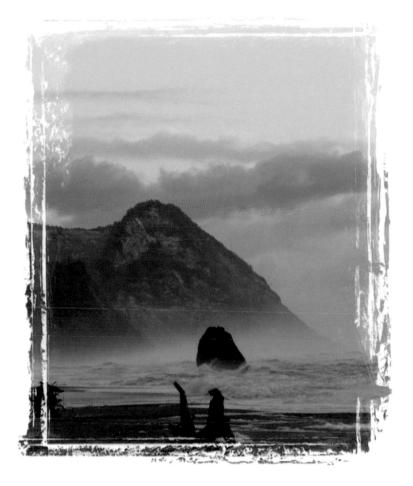

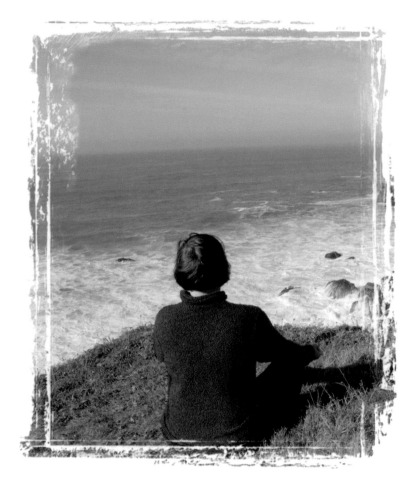

Be still and know that I am God.

CHAPTER 5

Learning to Surrender: Relaxation, Meditation, and Prayer

Everybody wants to feel good. We all want to feel safe and loved and accepted. And many of us have tried to find those feelings through inappropriate behaviors and addictions. When we see someone being compulsive, controlling, and self destructive, it's hard to remember that they are really trying to find peace, but most often, that is true. Nobody likes feeling uptight and tense. Nobody likes being in pain.

The 12-Step program asks us to turn our will and our lives over to the care of a Higher Power. This process is called surrender. It is a solution that truly gives us the peace we seek. It is very simple, but not always easy. What is required is a complete willingness to trust and have faith.

Learning to surrender has been a difficult process for me. I often find myself resisting and holding onto my defenses, rather than yielding to the circumstances of my life with trust and faith. And so I think about surrender every day. When I awake each morning I remind myself to stay open to the mystery of life without trying to control, fix, or force things to happen my way. I remind myself again and again to let go of struggle, resistance, and fear. Yielding and receptivity are the qualities I seek.

One of the things that helps me to surrender is taking time each day to still my body and quiet my mind. The techniques offered in this chapter — relaxation, meditation, and prayer — are the tools I use to get in touch with my inner guidance. As I learn to relax and simply stay receptive, I become conscious of an intuitive knowing that is somehow linked to my Higher Power. This inner voice can guide me in my life decisions if I listen. Learning to listen begins with trusting that there is indeed a loving presence guiding my life. I do not always feel this presence. And I certainly don't always feel surrendered. But when I take time for relaxation, meditation, and prayer I do begin to feel at peace. I actually feel a calming and healing energy rise up within me from the depths of my being. It is like opening a door to the grace of God, flowing through my life. That door is always there waiting to be opened, but I am so easily distracted. Our lives can get very busy. Yet when I allow myself to simply rest in stillness, even for a few moments, I am rewarded with clarity and ease. I am reminded of my desire to grow spiritually and my willingness to be open and receptive to life's lessons. This inward, quiet time helps remove my resistance to opening my heart and listening within. It helps awaken my faith with an inner consciousness that sees beyond the outer appearances of the world.

As you read through the following sections please realize that relaxation, meditation, and prayer are like any other learned skill: they get easier with practice. As we let go of our resistance to surrender, we welcome healing into our lives. As we align our will with that of a Higher Power, we find peace.

Relaxation

One of the nicest parts of yoga class is the relaxation period after practicing the postures. My students love this time, and so do I. It is a time to lie down in the Corpse Pose, allow your body to completely let go of all tension, and simply be. No doing, no performing. Just being.

Occasionally I have beginner students who have a difficult time letting go into relaxation. They do not know how to release the holding and tension in their bodies. Through yoga, they start becoming aware of tensions they never realized they had.

When this happens I think back to the first time I discovered how much stored tension I carried in my own body. Change begins with awareness. Before you know that something is out of balance it is hard to make a change. I first became aware of my need for relaxation when I was seventeen and decided to take some massage classes offered at a local health club. The instructor asked me if I had ever had a professional massage; when I said no, he told me that getting one was a prerequisite for the class. He said, "You must know how to receive before you can give."

Being massaged was my first experience of getting in touch with my body. That first massage gave me an awareness of how much tension I was holding. The therapist working on me kept telling me to let go and relax. But I had no idea of how to do that. I was still living with my parents at the time and my home environment was stressful. My father was an alcoholic, and he was dying of cancer. I was accustomed to living with a high level of stress and carrying accumulated tension in my body and mind, so much so that I did not even notice it.

It's difficult to stay relaxed when you are living with an alcoholic. I began tensing my muscles whenever my father was drinking, which became more and more frequent as his cancer progressed. It became like second nature for me to feel tense, so much so that I wasn't even aware of it. But that doesn't mean it wasn't taking a toll on my body.

That first massage was an eye-opener. After another year, during which I left home for college, my father died, and I was faced with making choices for my future, I decided to go to massage school to learn more about helping my body relax. A few years later, I began my studies in Hatha yoga, which further enhanced my ability to release tension from my body and mind.

Relaxation is a skill that anyone can learn. It is something that I learned, and so can you. Just as we create tension in our bodies through holding in feelings and contracting our muscles, we can create relaxation in our bodies through expressing our feelings and relaxing our muscles.

ACoA meetings taught me how to express my feelings but they didn't show me how to relax my body. Learning to relax is not difficult, but it does require conscious effort and, as with any learned skill, it requires patience and practice.

Some people say, "Oh, I relax by watching TV," or "I relax on the golf course," but this is not the kind of relaxation I am talking about. The kind of relaxation we need in order to heal our bodies is a total relaxation of body, mind, and spirit. Total relaxation requires "being" rather than "doing." It is a period of rest and tranquility that creates a calming effect on the mind and releases tension from the body. Practicing complete relaxation for even ten minutes a day relieves fatigue, reduces stress, and revitalizes the body. It is a period of rejuvenation and replenishment.

This is different from sleep. During sleep, you do not necessarily let go of the tensions in your body. In fact, studies have shown that the muscles do not relax at all as you sleep: the amount of muscular tension you fall asleep with is the amount of muscular tension you wake up with. Even if you wake up feeling refreshed after a night's sleep, it does not mean that the accumulated tension of weeks and years has been washed away.

Relaxation is an acquired skill. Complete relaxation requires focusing on the body and mind to relieve tension and create a feeling of peace and ease. When practiced regularly, relaxation allows us to prevent the body from building up and accumulating tension. It gives us an awareness of where we are holding tension in our body and how to release that tension. Deep relaxation allows for greater receptivity to healing. Developing this skill is one of the safest and most effective ways to manage stress, relieve anxiety, ease pain, and regain peace of mind.

This chapter gives your three relaxation scripts to use. Read them over once before trying them. Then ask a friend to read a relaxation script to you while you are lying down, or better yet, tape your own voice and listen to it while you are in the corpse pose. The scripts should be read slowly and softly. If you like you can play some soft, soothing music in the background. Some suggestions for music and for pre-recorded relaxation's are in the back of this book.

Practicing Relaxation

Relaxation can be practiced whenever you have ten or fifteen minutes to lie down in a quiet place, but the ideal time is right after you have practiced your Hatha yoga postures because you have already begun to release tension in your joints and muscles through stretching your body. To practice Hatha yoga without relaxation would be like making a cake without the frosting. Relaxation helps to release tensions not only in your body but also your mind. It is a time to let go completely and relax both physically and mentally.

The basic position for practicing relaxation is lying down on your back. A warm soft blanket will improve your comfort and ability to relax in this position.

When you lie down start with your knees bent and your feet flat on the floor. It is important for your knees to be bent because it helps to properly align your lower back. Put a pillow under your knees and thighs so you are not using your muscles to keep your knees bent. If you want to lie flat, begin with your knees bent and extend your legs one at a time without arching your back off the floor. Allow your legs to separate slightly. Place your arms down at your sides, slightly away from your body with your palms face up. Pull your shoulders down toward your feet. Gently extend the curve of your neck so that your chin comes down slightly. Make sure your teeth are slightly parted so that your jaw is relaxed. Close your eyes.

Tensing-Relaxing Technique

◆ Begin taking some long deep breaths. After four or five breaths, bring your awareness down to your feet, curling your toes and flexing your feet. Hold this for three seconds and as you exhale, let go and relax your feet.

◆ Now bring your awareness to your legs. As you inhale, squeeze and tighten your legs. Hold this for three seconds; as you exhale, release and relax your legs. Take a deep breath and release.

♦ Bring your awareness to your buttocks. As you inhale, squeeze and tighten your buttocks. Hold this for three seconds; as you exhale, release and relax your buttocks. Take another deep breath and release further.

♦ Bring your awareness to your shoulders. As you inhale, tense your shoulders by pushing them up toward your ears. Hold this position for 3 seconds; As you exhale gently press your shoulder blades down to the floor, opening the chest. Then think of gently pulling your shoulder down, away from your ears and toward your feet. Take a deep breath and release.

♦ Now bring your awareness to your chest area. As you inhale, press your shoulder blades into the floor while lifting and tensing your chest. Hold this for three seconds; as you exhale, release your shoulder blades and relax your chest.

♦ Bring your awareness to your shoulders. As you inhale, gently press your shoulder blades down to the floor, opening the chest. Then think of gently pulling your shoulder down, away from your ears and toward your feet. Take a deep breath and release.

♦ Next, bring your awareness to your arms and hands. As you inhale, tighten your arms and squeeze your hands into fists. Hold this for three seconds. Exhale, release the arms, relax the hands, and allow them to lie with palms up like gloves lying on a table, empty and still.

♦ Now bring your awareness to your face. As you inhale, tighten your face, crinkle your forehead, clench your teeth, make a prune face. Hold this for three seconds. As you exhale, relax your face, release your jaw, and enjoy the tingling sensation of all the tension leaving your face.

♦ Continue taking deep long breaths, focusing on your exhalations and allowing your body to relax more and more.

Breathing-Relaxing Technique

♦ Play some calm, soothing music in the background. Lie down for relaxation. Close your eyes. Mentally scan your body for tension. Notice if your neck, shoulders, or back feel tense. Take your time. If you notice any tightness, do not judge it to be negative. Just notice where you are feeling tension. You are checking in with your body in a loving way.

♦ After you have scanned your entire body for tension, bring your awareness to your breath. Imagine that you are able to breathe into each part of your body, helping it to relax and open. Visualize the air you are breathing in traveling to each body part.

♦ Begin with your feet. As you inhale, visualize the air traveling all the way down to your feet, helping them relax. As you exhale, all tension leaves your feet.

♦ Inhale and visualize the air traveling to your legs. Your legs become warm and relaxed as you inhale. As you exhale, all tension leaves the legs.

♦ Work your way up the body. Each time you inhale, you breathe in relaxation. Each time you exhale, you release tension. Take as long as you want at each body part, breathing into the area and helping it to relax.

♦ If you come to an area that feels particularly tight, keep breathing into that area. Visualize the breath going straight to that area helping it to relax and open. With every exhalation, tension leaves your body.

♦ As you work your way up, your entire body opens and widens. Your breathing is slow and even. You are relaxed.

Relaxation Visualization Technique

Often when I am teaching yoga classes for recovering people I use visualizations during the relaxation period which are designed to help my students in recovery. The following visualization script on self-love is an example.

♦ Lie down on your back. Start with your knees bent and your feet flat on the floor, gently pressing your lower back into the floor. Place a pillow under your knees for support or, if you want to lie flat, extend your legs one at a time without arching the back off the floor. Allow the legs to separate slightly.

♦ Place your arms down at your sides, with palms faced up in an attitude of receiving the life energy that circulates in the air around us. Make sure your teeth are slightly parted so that your jaw is relaxed. Relax your shoulders down toward your feet. Close your eyes.

♦ Start taking some deep, long breaths. Breathing in peace and relaxation. Exhaling and releasing all tension, all anxieties. Continue taking deep, long breaths. Your arms and legs are warm and heavy... warm and heavy. You are allowing yourself to relax.

- Using your breath and your thoughts to nurture yourself. Silently saying to yourself, *"I love and accept myself exactly as I am right now."* *"I love and accept myself exactly as I am right now."*
- Breathing in acceptance. Exhaling and releasing all self-criticism.
- Breathing in love. Exhaling and releasing all self-hate, all self-judgment.
- Allowing yourself to open and receive. All fatigue is leaving. Your body energy flows freely and evenly.
- Silently say to yourself, *"I allow myself to relax completely."* *"I allow myself to relax completely."* Feel your body opening and releasing all tension as it relaxes. The floor beneath you is supporting you completely. You are relaxed.
- Now visualize a warm, healing light shining above your body. This warm healing light is shining down on your body, sending love and warmth, sending healing energy to every atom and every cell in your body. And all you have to do is allow yourself to receive.
- Breathe in the light. This warm, healing light is calming and healing your entire body. Continue taking deep long breaths.
- Breathing in honesty. Exhaling and releasing all denial.
- Breathing in trust and faith. Exhaling and releasing all fear.
- Breathing in forgiveness for yourself and others. Exhaling and releasing all guilt and all resentment. Completely letting go.
- Allowing yourself to open, to expand, to surrender. Allowing yourself to receive. Allowing yourself to completely relax. To heal. To nurture yourself with deep breathing and positive thinking.
- Silently affirm to yourself, *"I am worthy of healing."* *"I am worthy of healing. I deserve to be well."* Give yourself permission to feel the ocean of love that is within you.
- Breathing in. Breathing out. Breathing in. Breathing out.
- Letting go completely. Resting.

Ending the Relaxation Period

Always come out of relaxation slowly; never jump right up. Begin by bringing your awareness back to your body. Become aware of the room around you. Without losing the feeling of quiet and calm that you have found, start to move and stretch.

Take your time. Begin by gently moving your fingers and your toes. When you feel ready, gently roll to one side, with your knees bent. Rest there for a moment. Then place your hand on the floor for support and gently sit up. Whenever possible, follow the relaxation period with meditation practice.

Meditation

Anyone working a 12-Step program knows that the eleventh step encourages us to improve our conscious contact with God through prayer and meditation. Yoga practice encourages us to do the same thing.

Meditation did not come easy for me. The first yoga class I ever took was given at Ananda Meditation Retreat in Nevada City, California. We began class with a half-hour session of postures. This was followed with some chanting and prayer to prepare us for meditation. The instructor informed us that we would sit in meditation for one hour.

I had never practiced meditation, so I was not quite sure of what to do. Everyone around me became quiet and still, with their eyes closed. I followed their example: I closed my eyes and sat there in silence. Every once in a while I opened my eyes to take a peek at what the others were doing. Everyone seemed to be in deep meditation. No one moved and no one seemed uncomfortable. They all sat there, perfectly still with their eyes closed.

I, on the other hand, was feeling very uncomfortable. My body began to hurt from holding it upright while sitting in one position for so long. I began to notice how stiff and tight my back and neck felt. When I tried to shift my weight, my movement seemed too loud. And my mind wandered in hundreds of directions. I wanted to get up and leave the room, yet I did not want to disturb the others or call attention to myself.

When the meditation finally ended, I spoke with the instructor about my experience. What I learned was that during that first hour, I was not meditating. I was not using a method to focus my mind or to quiet it. I was not even observing my thoughts. I just let them run wild and felt miserable sitting there. It was a long hour.

Meditation itself is a state of mind. It entails quieting the mind, emptying it out, letting go of all the chattering and racing thoughts. It is a calm, quiet state where there is no worry or confusion. When the mind is quiet, we become an open channel to our Higher Power. It is said that prayer is for talking to God and that meditation is for listening.

There are various methods for attaining a state of meditation. You can begin by having one point of attention to focus on, such as sitting and gazing at a candle flame, or sitting with your eyes closed and repeating an affirmation such as "peace" or "relax" silently to yourself each time you exhale. You can also simply focus on the breath itself, watching as it flows in and out. The idea is to keep your attention on the point of focus. No matter what comes up in your mind, notice it honestly without judgment and then go back to the point of focus.

It is interesting to watch what thoughts arise from the mind. At first there are many: "I feel silly sitting here, I wonder what I should have for dinner tonight, I do not like the neighbor's fence,…" So many thoughts. Each time I catch my mind chattering while I am meditating, I remind myself to focus again on the candle flame or on my breath or on whatever my point of focus is. It is an exercise in concentration. The process sometimes gets frustrating, but frustration is just one more thought. In time, the mind will stay quiet for longer and longer periods. Just keep bringing your attention back.

It helps to sit in a position that keeps your spine in a straight line while meditating. This keeps your energy moving upward. If you slump over or lie down, you may fall asleep. Meditation is not sleep. It is a state of relaxed alertness, a quiet awareness between the conscious and subconscious mind. Many people sit on pillows or folded blankets with their legs crossed or in a supported kneeling position. A chair is okay as long as you sit up straight, with your feet flat on the floor.

For many people, the purpose of Hatha yoga is to prepare the body for sitting in meditation. It is hard to sit still for any length of time if your body is stiff, tense, or uncomfortable. After doing postures, it is much easier to sit with the spine relaxed and erect for long periods of time.

I usually meditate twenty minutes a day. It's enough for me, although some people sit longer. I'm not always consistent. I've found that it's easier for me to meditate when I am with others and it is a shared activity. Many communities offer classes in meditation, and this is a good way to get started. If you are new to meditation, working with a teacher is advised.

I begin and end my meditations with prayer. The Serenity Prayer is my favorite, but sometimes I simply ask to be shown God's will, since control is something I have a difficult time letting go of. I always have to remind myself there is a Higher Power guiding my life, and I don't have to control or fix things. As I surrender to my Higher Power I am given the guidance I need to follow my own life path. Meditation helps me surrender.

To practice meditation, try any of the following techniques.

Candle Gazing: An Exercise in Concentration

- Find a warm, quiet, dark room. Place a lighted candle in the room so that you can sit and watch the flame. The candle should be at eye level about three feet (1 metre) away from you.
- Gaze at the flame without blinking for a minute or two. When your eyes begin to water, close them and visualize the candle flame in your mind. As the image starts to fade, open your eyes again and gaze at the candle flame.
- As thoughts come up in your mind, keep bringing your attention back to the candle flame. If your eyes water after a short time, simply close them again and visualize the flame in your mind's eye until the image vanishes. With practice you will gradually be able to extend the period of gazing. As your concentration goes deeper, your gaze will become steadier. In time you will be able to visualize the candle flame quite easily when you close your eyes.

Silent Word Repetition

- Sit in a comfortable position with your spine straight.
- Close your eyes and begin by paying attention to your breathing. Inhale slowly and deeply. As you exhale, silently and slowly say the word "peace" with the exhalation.
- Visualize the word "peace" written in front of you. Inhale deeply, and again as you exhale silently think "peace."
- If your mind wanders keep bringing it back to the word "peace." Keep coming back to your breathing. As your mind becomes still, your breathing continues to be slow and even. Remain motionless in this position for as long as is comfortable, becoming more and more aware of what is occurring within.
- Other words that can be used are love, patience, joy, forgiveness, trust, and relax.

Sitting in Silence

Sometimes simply sitting in silence is healing in itself. In this practice, you bring your attention to the sounds of silence. This may include sounds of nature: the Earth, the wind, the rain, the stillness of night-time. If you are indoors, you might become extremely aware of a clock ticking, which you had not noticed before. Use whatever sounds you find as a focal point for your mind. Ideally, it is best to find a place and time away from activity and noise. If you live in a city, it can be helpful to spend five or ten minutes sitting in silence, perhaps in the early morning as the sun is rising or late at night when things have settled down.

Our modern world is filled with noise pollution which hinders the sounds of the natural world — traffic, television, vacuum cleaners, lawn mowers ... the list goes on and on. Some people never experience the natural sounds of nature and silence. And yet silence is soothing to our nervous system. Making a conscious effort to be in silence is healing, even if it is done with earplugs.

Journal Entry

My name is Teresa. I am a child of an alcoholic. I am also a child of God. I have struggled many years to find a place of peace and acceptance. I have sought outside myself, reaching for alcohol and food, relationships and drugs, to fill the vast emptiness and to cover the pain within. I have spent my life running from myself, not wanting to face the fear and self-loathing.

Yoga has brought me to my knees in prayerful meditation. Through great introspection I have discovered within myself a center of light that is wholly loving and wholly lovable. In this place of peace I am able to surrender my fear and anxiety to my Higher Power.

Discovering my spiritual center has been the most powerful healing process in my recovery. When I am caught up in the daily struggle with my ego I can simply close my eyes, breathe deeply and know that in this very moment I am a peaceful, loving person. I am grateful that I was guided to yoga and meditation as a means of helping me in my recovery.

Teresa *(Recovering Adult Child)*

Prayer

Prayer is a powerful practice. The moment of prayer is always an event. It is an action of recognition and honor to the invisible forces that guide our lives. As a spiritual practice, prayer works. It may work in an entirely different way than we think, and it may be that we do not recognize the answers when they come. But when we pray, answers do come. Many times prayer appears to have failed because we ask for what we want of our own will rather than that of a Higher Power.

Step eleven suggest that we pray for two things and two things only: The knowledge of God's will for us and the power to carry it out. With prayer we surrender to the wisdom of a Higher Power.

Many people only pray when they are facing a crisis — "Oh God, please help me!". But prayer is not a cry to be used only in emergencies. It is not a plea to be rescued. It is not a time to make deals with God: "I'll change my ways if you get me out of this". These are dysfunctional forms of prayer based on fear rather than faith.

Healthy prayer is the voice of faith and love. It is a giving out, an offering. Through prayer we acknowledge and express our heartfelt desire to receive guidance and protection from God. As we offer our will and the care of our lives over to a Higher Power, we become vessels for divine inspiration and service to others. In this way prayer is healing. It is a lifeline that links us to a higher consciousness and unites us with humanity in a spiritual way.

When I pray I simply ask for clarity and guidance. I also find something in my life to be grateful for and I give thanks. This is not always easy, especially if I am feeling confused and overwhelmed. But if I allow my mind to be open I can always find something to be grateful for: often it is the beauty of nature or a friend in my life, or my health. Thanking my Higher Power for the abundance I have reminds me to keep faith in the midst of my confusion. It helps me to stay open and to be patient, knowing that clarity and guidance will come in time.

Prayer offers direct communication to God as we understand Him. It helps us acknowledge God's presence in our lives. When we call upon God we become humble. We open ourselves to discovering our deepest hopes and fears and to experience our childlike innocence. With our own stubborn willpower out of the way we can allow the grace of God to enter our lives.

When I introduce prayer in my yoga classes, each student's faith is supported. Prayer is a personal practice. Through prayer we make a connection with a Higher Power however we may conceive of or visualize it. For some, it may be praying to God, Christ, Buddha, Mother Mary, a Great Master, or to angels and guides. Whatever faith and form we choose, prayer is an offering, a giving of ourselves.

On the next pages you will find prayers from a variety of traditions.

THE SERENITY PRAYER

God, grant me the serenity to accept the things I cannot change,
the courage to change the things I can,
and the wisdom to know the difference.

THE LORD'S PRAYER

Our Father who art in heaven — hallowed be thy name.
Thy kingdom come, thy will be done,
On Earth as it is in heaven.
Give us this day our daily bread; and forgive us our debt
As we forgive our debtors.
And lead us not into temptation, but deliver us from evil.
For thine is the kingdom, and the power, and the glory
forever and ever.
Amen.

PRAYER OF ST. FRANCIS

Lord, make me an instrument of thy peace:
where there is hatred — let me sow Love;
where there is injury — Pardon;
where there is doubt — Faith;
where there is despair — Hope;
where there is darkness — Light;
where there is sadness — Joy.
O divine Master,
grant that I may not so much seek to be consoled, as to console;
to be understood, as to understand;
to be loved, as to love.
For it is in giving that we receive;
it is in pardoning that we are pardoned;
it is in dying that we are born to eternal Life.

PSALM 116

I love the Lord because He hears my prayers and answers them.
Because He bends down and listens, I will pray as long as I breathe.

SENECA PRAYER

Oh, Great Mystery —
Grant that I walk
A path with heart
Forever in balance and harmony.

LOVING KINDNESS PRAYER

May I be at peace.
May my heart remain open.
May I be awakened to the light of my true nature.
May I be healed.
May I be the source of Healing for all Beings.

SIOUX PRAYER

Grandfather, great Spirit
fill us with the Light;
give us the strength to understand
and the eyes to see.
Teach us to walk the soft Earth as relatives to all that live.

UNTITLED

Oh Great Lord,
may we know thee more clearly,
Love thee more dearly,
Follow thee more nearly,
for ever and ever
Amen.

PRAYER OF COMPASSION

May all beings be free from suffering.
May all beings be at peace.
May all beings be healed.
May all beings be happy.
May all beings be at peace.

AN IRISH BLESSING

May the road rise up to meet you,
May the wind be always at your back,
May the sun shine warm upon your face,
And the rains fall soft upon your fields,
And until we meet again,
May God hold you in the palm of His hand.

PRAYER OF MOTHER TERESA

Make us worthy, Lord, to serve our fellow men
throughout the world who live and die in poverty and hunger.
Give them through our hands this day their daily bread,
and by our understanding love, give peace and joy.

Journal Entry

When I am still I remember that inside of me is a place of calmness and love. I find this place in meditation. It is not always easy to find because I have built up many walls in my life. I have layers of resistance and fear. I have confused feelings inside of anger, sadness, resentment, and guilt.

But when I allow myself to relax and go inside, I find that underneath all the waves of emotions and feelings is a place of peace and acceptance. It's like there is some part of me, which I call my Higher Power, that knows how to trust the circumstances in my life without worry or fear.

I like the yoga affirmation: "Serenity comes when I surrender." Yoga prepares me for sitting quietly. prayer helps me be open and receptive. Meditation gives me surrender.

Lisa *(Recovering Addict)*

Journal Entry

I am not by nature an introspective person. Meditation, slowing down to go inside, does not come easy to me. I love the state "slowing down my mind" brings to me (or brings me to), I just don't very often get there.

In Annalisa's yoga class I manage to obtain that state of quiet clarity. A synergy exists in her work where the sum (and end) is much more than the parts. Stretching, breathing, relaxing, massage, guided visual- ization — each component feeds the others.

True healing takes place simultaneously on many levels. Mental/emo- tional healing occurs via affirmations. Somatic or body healing comes through stretching and massage; and cellular, deep healing occurs as you breathe. Yet the real power of the program lies in the way music, move- ment, stillness, affirmation, and group mind all contribute to the whole.

After a session I feel cleansed, calm, alert, and quiet. This is what people who meditate describe.

Dave *(Recovering Addict)*

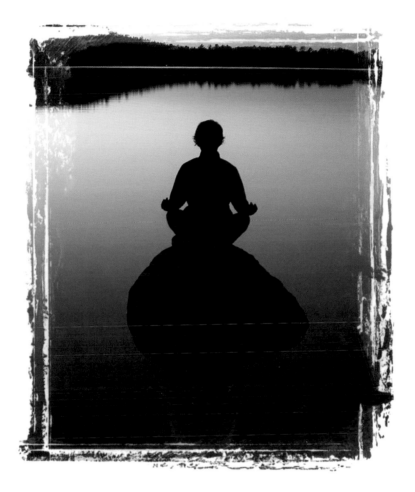

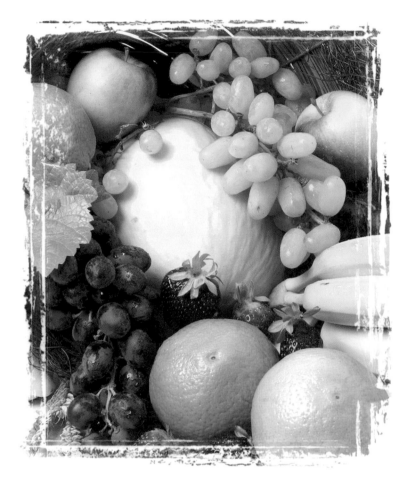

Keep it simple.

CHAPTER 6

Eating well is part
of Loving Yourself

For many years I used food as a means to cover up my feelings and fill the emptiness I felt inside. When I felt anxious, depressed, or out of control I would eat. Rather than allow my feelings to surface I tried to stuff them back down with food. Because of this I was overweight. When I looked in the mirror I was unhappy so I began counting calories. I tried various diets, always vowing to lose weight and always failing. I began to understand why the word "diet" contains the word "die." Each time I failed to stick to a diet, my belief in myself would die.

When I began studying Hatha yoga, I was introduced to the idea of eating food to improve health and vitality. I learned that some foods give me more energy and others actually deplete my energy. I was in my early twenties at the time and was very self-conscious about my weight. There is a great amount of pressure in our culture to look and stay thin. I remember thinking of food in terms of calories and weight loss rather than vitamins, minerals, and enzymes that nourish me. I tried various diets, always vowing to lose weight and always failing. I was perhaps 5-8 pounds heavier than my ideal weight, but my desire to be thinner was on my mind all the time.

Yoga taught me to view food in a different way. I learned which foods help heal the body and which foods have a negative effect and place stress on the system. Because I was also learning to reduce stress through stretching, breathing, and relaxation, I did not have an urge to eat when I was not hungry. As my body became healthier, I began to actually crave the foods that were healthy for me; non-nutritious filler foods were no longer appealing. Without trying, I began to lose weight. I also began to have more energy and vitality.

Most yogis advocate a vegetarian diet of pure, fresh, natural foods. The closer a food is to its natural state – fresh, unfrozen, unprocessed, and unrefined – the better it is for you. Just as prana life energy is in the air we breathe, it is also in the food we eat. Food that is high in prana is fresh, pure, natural, nutritional food. The yogic way of eating is natural and compassionate. Yoga offers diet recommendations that are designed to keep our bodies functioning at their best, give us the most energy, and contain the fewest toxins.

Also, each person is unique. People with specific food allergies need to adjust their diet choices to their body chemistry and condition. Diet is a very individual matter, yet all of us can bring conscious awareness to improve our eating habits. This is one more way to nurture ourselves and enhance health. Eating nutritious foods can help reduce stress and allow the body to repair and strengthen its natural defenses against disease. With healthy eating habits, we gain more energy, vitality, strength, and endurance.

As you read through this chapter, I ask you to keep an open mind. The dietary changes I advocate do not have to be made all at once. Gradual changes are often more permanent than those that happen overnight. Recovery is a process. Eating well is one more step in the recovery process which indicates that you are taking care of yourself and that you value yourself. Eating well is a part of loving yourself.

Unhealthy Habits

The first Al-Anon meeting I went to had coffee and doughnuts in the back of the room. I walked in and saw several people reach for a cup of coffee before the meeting began. I did the same. After the meeting some of the members introduced themselves to me. I spent a few minutes talking with them while having more coffee and a doughnut.

I appreciate those people and that first meeting enormously. Being there was the beginning of my life in 12-Step recovery. But after having coffee and a doughnut, my body did not appreciate the quick rise in blood sugar which was inevitably followed by a steep drop. Sugar and caffeine are stressors to the body and mind. These substances dramatically change our blood sugar levels and throw our body chemistry out of balance. Usually, once the blood sugar has dropped there is a craving for more sugar and/or caffeine to spike it back up again. These fluctuating blood sugar levels can cause moodiness, depression, irritability, anxiety, and fatigue. And so the roller coaster ride begins.

I believe that sugar and caffeine are just as addictive as alcohol. In small amounts they may do no harm, if you are healthy. If your health is compromised, these substances will add additional stress to your system. Those of us who are recovering from compulsive or addictive behavior should be aware of how much and how often we use these substances. Moderation is not one of our strong points. Sugar and caffeine not only unbalance our body chemistry and increase our level of stress, they also offer no nutritional value. In fact, caffeine actually draws B vitamins out of the body. Sugar and caffeine reduce our body's ability to fight stress and to heal.

If your health is compromised in any way then I suggest you eliminate sugar and caffeine from your diet. You may be surprised at how much more energy you have for healing once you get through the initial withdrawal from cravings. If you need medical support while quitting these substances, I suggest you find a nutritional doctor in your local area. Nutritional medicine is a speciality in and of itself, with many excellent practitioners who can guide you.

Stopping or reducing your intake of sugar or caffeine is not always easy, especially if you have become addicted. You may experience some withdrawal symptoms if you quit cold turkey. If you can work a 12-Step program for that, then go for it. Make sure you have a network of other recovering people who also have a desire to quit using sugar or caffeine. Read labels and notice how many foods contain these substances. If you don't feel ready or willing to give up sugar and caffeine completely then work on reducing your intake.

I suggest that you start by replacing sugar with fresh fruit. Whenever you get a craving for something sweet try eating an apple. Apples are easy to take along with you wherever you go. At first you may feel deprived of those sweets you love but your mind will soon adapt as you become calmer, clearer, and healthier. When this happens your cravings for sugar will decrease.

As for caffeine, there are plenty of decaffeinated coffees and beverages available. I struggle with this addiction myself. I often start my day with a cup of coffee. I enjoy the flavor. I like the lift that coffee gives me, and when I travel I enjoy buying speciality coffees to bring home with me. Caffeine is a very popular drug worldwide, perhaps the most popular. Although I have a habit of drinking coffee, I limit my intake. I do not drink more than two cups per day. And I pay attention to my energy levels. If I am sick or feeling fatigued and stressed, I stop drinking coffee completely until I feel better again. I want to give my body all the energy it needs for healing.

Each time I quit drinking coffee I feel sluggish for a few days as the caffeine is leaving my system, but afterwards I feel renewed energy and calmness of mind. My energy is stable rather than stimulated. I also notice that I am more in tune with my feelings and my intuition. Coffee has a tendency to gear me up.

The high I get from caffeine stimulates my thoughts, but can also take me away from my feelings. Sound familiar?

I have managed to go without coffee for months at a time, but somehow the opportunity to enjoy just one cup with friends has always lured me back into a daily habit. Thus for me, it is indeed an addiction. Perhaps one day I will quit forever.

If you have a weakness for sugar or caffeine then pay attention to your energy levels. Observe how these substances affect your overall feeling of well being. When you first eat sugar or drink caffeine your blood sugars will rise quickly, stimulating your energy. But after a short while your blood sugars fall and you feel tired, often craving more sugar or caffeine. To avoid this up and down addictive cycle we need to eat healthy food in healthy amounts, which will keep our blood sugars stable.

More About Blood Sugar

Because stabilizing blood sugar levels is important for reducing stress I want to explain further what blood sugar is and how it works in our bodies.

Simply defined in the dictionary, blood sugar is the glucose in the blood that rises and falls depending upon what you eat. All carbohydrates are ultimately converted to glucose to be used by the body as fuel for the brain and muscles. That's why when we are feeling low on energy we often crave sugar or caffeine (caffeine appears to release stored glucose). We instinctively know that these substances will raise our energy (or sugar level) very rapidly. The problem is that this high concentration overloads the system, causing the levels to spike way above normal and then fall rapidly to way below normal. Then we feel even more tired and crave more sugar… so then we spike again....crash again...over and over. This chemical roller coaster ride can cause irritability, depression, confusion, anxiety, and fatigue. It's just another addiction cycle. Not only are the symptoms unpleasant on their own, they also often lead to relapse into other unhealthy addictions. And so the vicious cycle of not taking care of ourselves continues.

To avoid this up and down addictive cycle we need to eat healthy food in healthy amounts. Ideally we want a steady, strong level of energy all day long. This is achieved by avoiding sugar and caffeine, and instead eating whole foods that are digested slowly, such as the complex carbohydrates (fruits, vegetables, grains). There is more information about which foods are healthy to eat later in this chapter.

Understanding blood sugar levels is particularly helpful to those of us who have lived with alcoholics or are recovering from alcoholism. The high sugar content of alcohol (and the spikes and crashes of blood sugar that result) has a lot to do with the mood swings that alcoholics are known for. There is also a definite connection between sugar addiction and alcohol addiction — and it is easy to go from one to the other.

Fast Food Is Dead Food

One of the first rules of nutrition I learned when I began studying Hatha yoga was: "Do not eat dead foods." At first, I did not know what that meant. I had never thought about food as being alive; I certainly had not thought that some foods had more life than others. Then it was pointed out to me that foods with life energy are the foods that give life energy to me. They give me the nutrients my body needs.

Dead foods are those foods that have been robbed of their natural vitamins, minerals, amino acids, and enzymes due to processing. They include canned, preserved, bleached, polished, refined, and otherwise devitalized foods.

Oftentimes these dead foods are presented to us as fast foods and convenience foods. They are called convenient because they are easy to prepare and they save us time. Just open a can or take a package out of the freezer, heat it up and in 10 minutes you have a meal.

If you have not eaten at home, you can always grab a quick bite to eat at a nearby fast-food restaurant. Television commercials advertise the fun and convenience of ordering a pizza or enjoying a burger and fries with our loved ones. The advertisements do not mention the nutritional value of such food, perhaps because there is none. Fast foods are generally refined – high in fat, sugar, and salt – and nutrient-poor. Although they may work just fine to soothe your appetite, they do little to give you the necessary vitamins, minerals, amino acids, and enzymes that your body needs. They do little to build and maintain a healthy body.

Foods for Reducing Stress and Building Health

Fruits and Vegetables

Eat lots of fresh fruits and vegetables. Make a big green salad with a variety of raw vegetables as part of your daily diet — it's excellent for your health. Raw vegetables contain plenty of nutrients and fiber that your body needs. Cooked vegetables are also fine as long as they are not overcooked, so that all the vitamins and minerals are lost. Ask for lightly steamed vegetables whenever possible. Baked carrots, squash, and potatoes are also very good (and when you've been off sugar for a while, they taste really sweet), it's what we put on top of them that hurts us: sugar, butter, and sour cream.

Avoid canned fruits and vegetables because these are often "dead" foods that contain added sugar and salt. Sea vegetables such as kelp, nori, and kombo are excellent mineral sources and taste great when added to soups. They can usually be found in health food stores.

Vegetable Juices

Fresh vegetable juices are a good source of enzymes, minerals, and other nutrients. Buying a juicer is a worthwhile investment. You can have juice several times a day, as a between-meal snack or with a meal. For best results, consume the juice within 15 minutes of juicing the vegetables. Because carrot juice can raise your blood sugar, dilute it in half with green vegetable juice or water.

Organic Produce: Is It Worth It?

Organically grown foods are those produced without chemical fertilizers or pesticides. Most farms are required to farm organically for three years before the food they produce can be labeled "certified organic." This allows time for the soil to be remineralized and for harmful chemicals to be removed. The popularity of organic produce is growing rapidly as people begin to recognize the harmful effects of the huge amounts of pesticides sprayed on farmland each year. The consumption of organic products can reduce the risks of chemical exposure, both to individuals and to the planet. Organic foods are not only free of chemical residue, but they taste better and have many more nutrients than commercially farmed foods.

To help improve your health and the health of the environment buy organic, local, and seasonal produce whenever possible. The more we support organic farmers, the less pesticides are produced. I have heard some people complain that organic food is more expensive and that they cannot afford the extra cost. I say you cannot afford not to make sure you are eating nontoxic foods. You are worth the extra cost. It is an investment in your health and your planet.

Whole Grains and Legumes

Gradually reduce and eliminate refined foods from your diet. These include white sugar, white flour, white bread, white rice, and white pasta products. Eat whole grains instead. Look for products such as whole-wheat or rye flour, multigrain breads and cereals, brown rice, oats, millet, and buckwheat. Once you make up your mind to stop eating refined foods, you will find lots of options available. You may have to adjust at first to new textures and tastes, but remember that refined foods have been stripped of important nutrients and fiber. Even though they taste good, they place more stress on your system.

Whole grains are rich in B-complex vitamins, which play an essential role in keeping stress levels down. Whole grains also supply important amino acids to the body, especially when eaten with legumes. Combinations such as beans and rice or rice and lentil soap make great meals.

Nuts and Seeds

Nuts and seeds are healthy snack foods, especially if eaten raw. These foods are good sources of protein, but are also high in oils, so if you are on a fat-restricted diet you will need to limit your intake. Avoid roasted nuts that have been heavily salted.

Adding nuts and seeds to your meals is fun and nutritious. Unhulled sesame seeds are high in calcium and taste delicious when sprinkled on grains. Sunflower seeds, pumpkin seeds, and almonds are great in salads or eaten alone.

I like to take a handful of almonds with me in my pocket when I know I will be having a busy day and will need extra energy. If I am working long hours and cannot take the time to have a complete meal, I can eat a few almonds throughout my day to keep my blood sugar from dropping. This is really important because low-blood-sugar cravings often result in bingeing and overeating.

Water

Water is one of the essential compounds of our body chemistry. An insufficient intake of water is often responsible for constipation, liver and kidney malfunctions, congested colon, and poor cell functioning. The only way to allow the body's sophisticated filtration system to work properly is to take in enough water to flush out the toxins that build up. For people detoxing from alcohol or substance abuse this is especially important.

You should drink at least six 8-oz. (0.25 liters) glasses of water every day. This is in addition to whatever other beverages you drink. Pure water helps your body excrete toxins. Water also regulates your body temperature and transports nutrients throughout your system.

It is best to drink purified, spring, or distilled water. This is preferable to the processed, softened, or polluted tap water that is found in many communities.

Foods to Consider Reducing from Your Diet

Dairy Products

For years I ate dairy products as one of my main foods. I especially liked cheese. I also drank milk and used it on my cereals. In my early thirties, I developed allergies to various pollens and molds in the air. A friend suggested that if I stopped eating dairy products my allergies would get better because dairy products create mucus in the system. Because I was miserable, I tried following my friend's advice — and my allergies cleared up. You may want to try this experiment yourself.

Since that time I have eaten very little dairy. In place of milk, I use soy milk, which tastes great to me. I seldom eat cheese. If I do eat cheese, I make sure it is natural and not processed with added sugar, salt, and preservatives. Always read the labels. Soy cheeses are also available, although I have to admit that they do not taste good to me. However, I have friends who like soy cheese. You have to experiment for yourself. Limiting your cheese intake is a good idea because cheese is high in saturated fat and often high in salt. Low fat cheese such as cottage or ricotta is generally easier to digest and better absorbed than hard cheeses like swiss, cheddar, and parmesan. Lowfat milk is better than regular if you are going to drink milk.

Avoid common "processed cheeses" that come in boxes or pre-sliced (or that squirt out of a can!), they have added sugar, salt, and preservatives. Read labels and if you can't pronounce or recognize half the ingredients, think twice about eating it.

Butter and margarine are also products that should be reduced or eliminated from the diet. Butter is made from cream and is high in saturated fats. Keeping fat out of your diet is important for self care and for reducing the risk of heart disease. Margarine is made from liquid vegetable oils and is hydrogenated, a process which adds hydrogen to natural oils to make them solid. In other words, margarine is actually man-made saturated fat, although not as saturated as butter. But margarine contains artificial additives and preservatives. If it is a choice between the two I suggest using butter in very small amounts. Eliminating butter and margarine completely is ideal. Health food stores sell natural oil spreads that can be substituted for butter. Ghee is another product found in health food stores that is a healthy replacement for butter. It is best to use any butter replacements in small amounts also.

Yogurt is a good source of protein and contains friendly bacteria that aid in digestion and intestinal functions. Look for natural yogurt that does not contain added sugar and artificial flavorings. Remember: read labels.

Eggs

Everyone knows that eggs are a good source of protein. Years ago I raised my own chickens and discovered the difference between fresh eggs and store-bought eggs. Fresh eggs definitely taste better. Although I seldom eat eggs these days, when I do I look for fresh brown eggs. Health food stores usually carry them and get them locally.

It is best to eat eggs that have been poached or boiled rather than fried in oil or scrambled in butter. Fried foods of any kind are hard on the digestive system. When I think of eating fried foods I think of eating grease. I imagine a pile of grease sitting in my stomach — not a pleasant thought. With that thought in mind, french fries and doughnuts no longer have much appeal. Neither do fried eggs. Eggs are high in cholesterol and should be avoided if that is a concern. Tofu can be used as an egg replacement for scrambled eggs.

Meat

There was a time when cows, pigs, sheep, chickens, and turkeys were raised organically on farms. They had healthy, natural lives. But these days the meat and poultry industries keep these animals locked up in crowded factories where they are severely mistreated and stuffed with chemicals, steroids, and antibiotics. After they are slaughtered, they are prepared with more additives and preservatives for our markets.

Because of this, many people avoid eating meat completely. If you choose to eat meat, look for meat that has been organically grown and is not filled with additives and preservatives. Processed meat such as bacon, ham, cold cuts, hot dogs, salami, and sausages contain numerous additives and are usually processed with some kind of sugar as a preservative. Read labels. Red meats such as beef and pork are high in saturated fat. Poultry and fish tend to be lower in saturated fats than other meats.

I cannot help thinking that spiritually we pay a price when we eat animals that have been kept in pain and terror throughout their lives. The grain that is used to feed and fatten livestock could feed five times the U.S. population. Hunger and malnutrition could be alleviated worldwide if we used that grain to feed people. Whether or not you agree with this view, it does merit some thought.

General Rules for Eating

- Eat slowly. Chew your food thoroughly. Digestion begins in the mouth.
- Allow time for your food to digest. Eating your meals in a relaxing environment without external distractions enhances your body's ability to digest and assimilate food effectively. Often people eat on the run; it is common to see people gulping down food as they rush off to work. This does not make for good digestion. Nurture yourself by enjoying sit-down meals eaten in a calm environment. Take your time.
- Drink 6 to 8 glasses of pure water daily. It is best to drink fluids between your meals.
- If you snack, choose healthy foods. Keep an assortment of healthy snack foods readily available in case you feel hungry. Celery sticks, an apple, or a bag of almonds are examples of healthy snack choices that will help curb your appetite and give you the added benefit of proper nutrition.
- Make a habit of reading the labels on foods. Avoid foods with additives, preservatives, and sugars.

Guidelines for Eating Well to Reduce Stress and Improve Health

Foods to Reduce or Eliminate

- Sugars and sweets: candy, ice cream, sugar-sweetened drinks, sugar-filled desserts, sugar coated cereals, and so on
- Caffeine: coffee, tea, cola, cocoa, and chocolates
- Refined foods (foods that contain additives and preservatives): sausages, bacon, cold cuts, hot dogs, salami, and so on
- Salt (causes fluid retention, high blood pressure, and heart disease)
- Canned foods (contain added sugar and salt)
- Condiments: mayonnaise, ketchup, pickles, and rich salad dressing (contain added sugar and salt)
- Meat and dairy products: look for organic and farm-raised if you can eat these.

Add and Enjoy

- Fresh fruits and vegetables (should make up 50–70% of your diet)
- Whole grains: brown rice, oats, millet, buckwheat, multigrain breads, and so on
- Legumes: peas, lentils, and beans
- Nuts and seeds (best eaten raw, unsalted, and in small quantities)
- Soy milk products (can replace diary products)
- Fresh fish (can replace meat)
- Herbal teas: peppermint, apple cinnamon, chamomile, and so on
- Water (at least six 8-oz. (0.25 liters) glasses a day)

What if You have No Choice?

Sometimes we are in situations where we have no choice about the food available for us to eat. For example, in hospitals, on airplanes, in jails, or in other institutions, your choice may be to eat what's offered or eat nothing at all. Most of the food that is offered in such places is refined and processed. In these situations it doesn't help to worry or be anxious about the sugar, fats, and additives you are ingesting. If you can't change your diet, change your attitude. Attitude can sometimes be more nourishing than food. You could be eating the healthiest foods in the world, but if you're thinking negatively while eating those foods you are still putting toxins into your system. For many people, the issues of food and diet bring up feelings of anger, worry, guilt, hatred, self-righteousness, obsessiveness, and rigidity. These are all pitfall attitudes that can sabotage the healthiest diet.

Whatever food you are eating, take time to bless it before you eat. This may sound corny but it's a great way to clear your attitude. When I take the time to bless my food it brings me to an attitude of thankfulness and gratefulness for what I have. Blessing my food reminds me to slow down and enjoy my meal in an unhurried manner rather than gobble it down quickly. When I eat slower I tend to eat less and I enjoy my food more.

Remember that feeding yourself is about loving yourself. Do the best you can to follow the guidelines for eating well to reduce stress and build health. If you find yourself eating junk food, don't beat yourself up with guilt. That's not loving yourself. Changing food habits is a process just like recovery. Take it one day at a time. Keep it simple and be gentle with yourself.

Journal Entry

The affirmation I concentrate on when doing yoga is "I am good to my body and my body is good to me." I am recovering from compulsive overeating. My food of choice was anything with sugar or chocolate.

With all the demands and stressors in life, I need to take time to nurture myself in positive ways instead of using food. Yoga has helped me to slow down and let go of certain feelings that may be the impetus in my overeating. I am learning to love myself more and to accept my flaws.

Food is slowly having a different meaning in my life. I am learning that nutritious food is important for my body and for my emotional health as well. When I eat healthy meals instead of bingeing on junk food I am less moody and my energy is more stable throughout the day.

As I slowly change my eating patterns I feel better about myself. Yoga helps me relax and gives me an opportunity to examine my thoughts and feelings. When I am relaxed I have less desire to overeat. When I am calm I make better choices in my life.

Lonna *(Recovering Compulsive Eater)*

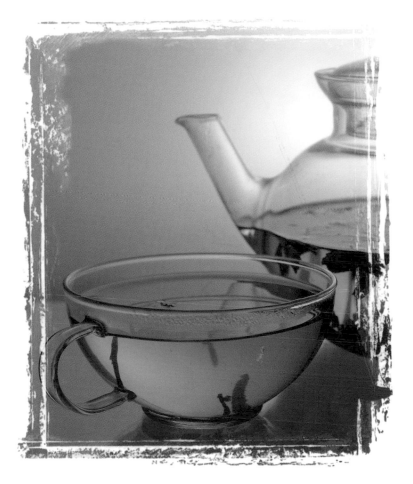

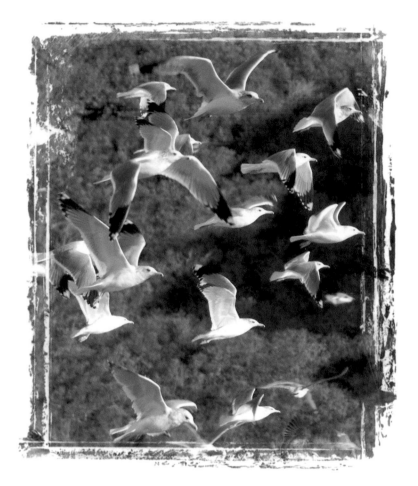

Allow aliveness to grow.

CHAPTER 7

Aerobic Exercise

When I was 22 years old, I went to Europe for the summer and traveled on a Eurail pass with a backpack, staying at youth hostels and camping outside. I did a lot of walking that summer and got into great physical shape.

When I got back to California at the end of summer, the friend I had left my car with told me the car was no longer running. The mechanic I took it to quoted me a thousand dollars to get the car fixed. I didn't have a thousand dollars. I had spent all of my money in Europe. Because I had no choice, I decided that I would live without a car for a while. "For a while" ended up being three years.

During that time, whenever I wanted to go somewhere I had four options: I could walk, I could ride my bicycle, I could bum a ride from a friend, or I could take the bus. Since I wasn't too good at asking for help in those days, I rarely got rides from other people. Occasionally I took the bus to travel long distances, but most of the time I rode my bike or I walked.

Living without a car was not always convenient. People used to ask me, "What do you do when it rains?" and I would simply answer, "I get wet." I had to learn to pace myself and allow plenty of time to get places. I had to learn to carry groceries in my bicycle basket, and buy small amounts at a time so I wasn't overloaded. I had to adjust to cold weather by wearing extra layers of clothes and rain gear. But the advantage of not having a car was that exercise was my lifestyle. I never thought about "getting my daily exercise", it just happened.

It is common knowledge that regular exercise improves our physical and mental well-being. Exercise helps burn calories, build and maintain muscle tone, improve circulation, and work the heart and lungs to keep them strong.

People often ask me if Hatha yoga is my only form of exercise. I answer that it is my favorite and most consistent form, but I also enjoy other aerobic activities, such as walking, swimming, bicycling, and dancing.

Aerobic exercise has become quite popular in the last 25 years. "Aerobic" refers to those activities that promote cardiovascular fitness by requiring the lungs and heart to use oxygen more efficiently. Any rhythmical activity that moves large muscle groups and elevates the heartbeat and respiratory rate for sustained periods of time is considered aerobic.

There are many reasons for the popularity of aerobic exercise. The development of self-esteem, feeling of accomplishment, and physical enhancement involved in both weight loss and muscle development are the obvious. But there are also subtle, unseen ways in which exercise can help us. It has been discovered through scientific research that sustained aerobic exercise actually increases the endorphin levels in the brain. Endorphins are tranquilizer-like neurochemicals which give us euphoric feelings and help with pain management.

In terms of addiction and recovery, this means that regular aerobic exercise may help alleviate drug cravings and depression. Knowing this, one might certainly recommend aerobic exercise to recovering people. There is danger in this, however. Those of us who are in recovery have a tendency to be compulsive. Compulsive exercise is like anything else we do compulsively: it is self-defeating. In the case of exercise, compulsiveness often leads to injury.

As you read through the various aerobic exercises discussed in this chapter, keep in mind the yogic approach to movement and the body. In Hatha yoga the movement is never forced. Every pose is gently directed and relaxed into. Rather than forcing performance and endurance, the body is encouraged to open, stretch, and strengthen at its own rate of surrender. The goal is not to push the body beyond its limits but rather to allow the body to grow in its natural capacities for flexibility, strength, and balance. Yoga teaches respect for the body.

Since I've been practicing Hatha yoga I've learned to use this same approach when participating in other forms of exercise. For instance, if I decide to go for a run with a friend, I listen to my body and run at a pace that I can handle. For me this is usually a slow jog or a fast walk, since I don't run often and have little endurance for it.

If you learn to approach exercise in a healthy way it can be a wonderful part of your recovery lifestyle. Becoming and remaining healthy means listening to your body. It means viewing your body as a friendly barometer. Take it slowly. If you begin an exercise program and find that you're feeling overly exhausted, immediately cut back on the exercise. If you find that a certain exercise makes your body hurt in general or causes you specific pain, stop doing that particular exercise. Treat your body gently, with care.

One way to avoid injury is to incorporate Hatha yoga postures into your exercise program. Exercise can take many forms but the most effective routines include a warm-up period, 20 to 30 minutes of elevated heart beat, and a cool-down at the end.

Warm-up means raising the body temperature and loosening the muscles in preparation for movement. Taking 10 or 15 minutes to breathe, stretch, and strengthen the muscles before you begin an aerobic activity is an ideal warm-up. Once you've finished your aerobic workout, it is beneficial to cool-down with 15 to 20 minutes of stretching and 10 minutes of relaxation. If you take the extra time to do this your body will be well-rewarded for the effort it put forth.

Any of the following aerobic activities can be adapted to follow the yogic principals of conscious breathing and awareness with movement; and these exercises can be valuable complements to your yoga practice.

Walking

Walking is one of the oldest and most natural forms of exercise. We are made to walk. Walking is an ideal exercise because it can be done virtually at any time and at any place. We can walk with others or alone, and walking is cost-free. It's also virtually injury-free. Walking places little stress on the bones and joints. People seldom get injured from walking.

If you are physically out of shape, walking is one of the easiest ways to begin an aerobic exercise program. Start out modestly, walking only a few blocks each day. As you become more fit you can walk longer distances.

The important thing for aerobic walking is to walk briskly. You must walk at a fairly fast pace the entire time without stopping to chat with other people. To prevent myself from the temptation to stop and talk with someone while I'm walking, I usually find a friend to walk with me. I've found that visiting friends while we walk together can be fun, and is often healthier than going out to lunch where we spend our time together sitting and eating.

To increase upper body movement and help raise your heart rate, you can swing your arms as you walk. I suggest doing what is comfortable for you. As you walk briskly your arms should swing naturally. As you build up strength and endurance, you may want to add more movement for the upper body.

In the beginning, stick to level ground. Walk for 30 minutes nonstop and notice how your body feels. As you get in shape and want a more challenging workout you can walk on uphill grades. You'll be surprised at how much endurance it takes to walk up hills.

I recommend making walking a part of your lifestyle the way I recommend yoga. Even if you don't use walking as your aerobic activity you can still improve your health simply by adding more walking to your life. There are various small ways that you can do this easily. For instance, when you drive some place and are looking for a parking spot, park your car a few blocks away from your destination. You'll get the benefit of walking — and it's usually easier to find a parking space! If you're in a building and you have a choice between riding in an elevator and taking the stairs, use the stairs. Every time you choose to use your legs you are exercising your body and improving your health. It doesn't take much to change sedentary living into healthy habits of movement. I encourage you to walk as often as possible. Walking is easy to incorporate into your daily life and beneficial for you.

Running

Several of my friends swear by running. I remember one friend told me that running was like getting high. Years later I learned that running releases endorphins and I finally understood what my friend was talking about. For him, running was a fix. The problem with this of course, is compulsiveness. I've known some people who were so compulsive about running that even when they had an injury they didn't stop. A pulled tendon or a torn ligament won't heal without rest.

You also risk injury if you get into running without taking appropriate precautions. While it's true that running is an easy and inexpensive way to get in shape and lose weight, it is also true that without proper care, running can be an easy way to injure the body.

It's a good idea, if you're going to take up running, to get a physical exam first. Even if you are physically fit, take it easy in the beginning, and increase your distance slowly. Most running injuries are the result of pushing beyond one's limit. Start your running program with a slow jog or even a fast walk. The idea is to get your heart rate up, not to win the race. Let your endurance build over time. Then, if you want to race, be sure to find someone knowledgeable about race training to work with. Otherwise, remember to run for enjoyment and exercise. Keep it simple. Take it easy.

I recommend running for 20 to 30 minutes, three to four times a week. To some people that won't sound like much. To others it will. But the message is that 20 minutes of an elevated heart beat is all that is required to satisfy our need for cardiovascular exercise. If you want to run more than that, be careful not to overdo it.

You should consider what kind of shoes you run in. Even though I don't run often I did invest in high quality running shoes. When I do run, I want the best support for my feet. Most athletic shoe stores will tell you which shoes are beneficial for running and why.

Where you run is another factor. It always surprises me to see people running along busy roads, breathing in exhaust fumes as the cars drive by. Also, I refuse to run on pavements. I don't like the hard landing my body receives on cement; it feels jarring to me. Where do you run then? Look for parks, fields, running trails, anywhere that is not paved. I especially enjoy running on the sand at the beach. If you decide that running is your thing and you use it wisely – which means not overdoing it – it can be a rewarding activity that is beneficial for your recovery and well-being.

Swimming

I have always enjoyed swimming. For some reason, water is a healing element for me. I get in water and I feel that my tensions are being washed away. Aerobic swimming requires a body of water long enough for swimming distance or laps. Most people think of swimming laps in a pool but I've also enjoyed aerobic swimming in rivers, lakes, and in the ocean. If it's warm outside and I'm near safe water I usually swim.

One of the nice things about water is floating. Water eliminates the weight-bearing stress on joints and bones we usually deal with when we exercise. Because of this we are less likely to get injured. We feel lighter and freer to move.

When we swim we use the resistance of water to help strengthen the muscles, and long swimming strokes to stretch them. Thus swimming is a balanced sport that gives us an overall body workout. Some people would disagree and say that swimming is primarily an upper-body sport, but we do use our legs to propel the body as we swim. I've found that if I do a few extra laps with a kickboard, I've worked my lower body as well as my upper.

Another advantage of swimming is that it helps us focus on using our breath succinctly and evenly as we move. I have already discussed the benefits of deep, even breathing in Chapter Three. Because of our connection with the breath as we swim, this exercise is both energizing and calming.

Disadvantages to swimming? Some people develop ear, eye and sinus problems which are aggravated by the water. Some people are afraid or just don't like the water. Finding a place to swim may be complicated, and after-swim grooming may take too long for your busy schedule.

If you decide swimming is for you, again, 20 to 30 minutes, several times a week, is the recommendation for your cardio-vascular workout. Many health clubs now provide indoor lap pools for people who want to swim all year.

Aerobic Dance Classes

Aerobic classes featuring rhythmic dancing to music have become widely popular and accepted as a "fun and demanding" workout. Demanding is a good word for it. Often these programs are more strenuous than running. Shin splints, pulled muscles, and lower-back ailments are common aerobic injuries. If you get into an aerobics class that involves fast movements with a lot of jumping on a hard floor know that it can have a jarring impact on the body.

The key to enjoying a safe aerobic dance workout is to find a teacher who is well-trained and educated in physiology and injury prevention. A good teacher will be aware that members of the group will be at different levels of proficiency, suppleness, and ability. A good teacher will also know the quality of surface you are dancing on and will modify the workout as needed. There should be frequent reminders to take things at your own pace, and frequent demonstration of low-impact variations. Low-impact movements are designed to minimize the wear and tear on the skeletal and muscular systems. Qualified instructors will also demonstrate how to take your own heart rate and will do so several times during the class to make sure you are not overworking yourself.

One of the problems when doing aerobic dance is that some instructors prefer music so loud that it overwhelms signals from the body. When my focus is on the music, I find myself trying to keep up with everybody else, and I end up moving faster than my body wants to go. In this way aerobic dance has an outward rather than inward focus. Because of this, when I do aerobic dance, it is important for me to balance it with my Hatha yoga practice so that I stay in touch with how my body is feeling.

If you choose aerobic dancing, select a teacher and group with great care. Look for a situation in which you are encouraged to do low-impact movement and where you feel comfortable going at your own pace. If you experience any soreness or pain during or after a workout, discuss this with the teacher. A qualified teacher will show you how to move so that you won't get injured. If excessive soreness or any inflammation occurs, it's a good idea to have it checked by a doctor. We have the tendency to continue on and hope the pain will go away. But let me say again that part of our recovery is learning to respect and take care of our bodies. Aerobic dancing can be a fun exercise if we participate in it safely with a skilled teacher.

Bicycling

Bicycling is considered an aerobic exercise as long as you cycle at a speed of about 15 miles per hour. It's also a great means of transportation and can easily be incorporated into anyone's life as a healthy way to get around. It can be worked into your commute to work, or it can be your weekend fun activity.

If you cycle for aerobic exercise you need to do so regularly (three or four times a week) and you need to exert yourself by picking up speed for about 20 or 30 minutes during the ride. It's nice to cycle this way, then return home and stretch and relax.

It's also nice to use your bike for short trips without worrying about speed or distance. Using your bike instead of your car is good for the environment and good for your body.

Other Activities

The activities I've mentioned in this chapter are just a few of the many cardiovascular exercise options available. Others include tennis, skiing, skating, racquetball, basketball, and soccer. There are many forms of exercise and whatever works for you is great. My purpose in this chapter is simply to encourage you to do some type of aerobic activity on a regular basis, in addition to practicing Hatha yoga.

By the way, some forms of yoga are aerobic. Vinyasa yoga, meaning yoga that "flows together" incorporates a series of postures using salutations with pushups and jumps in-between to create an aerobic workout. Some people refer to this style as Power Yoga or Ashtanga yoga. Kundalini yoga also incorporates flowing movement with a breathing technique called "breath of fire" that can help raise the heart rate. And Bikram yoga offered in a heated room incorporates movement which helps raise the body temperature and makes a person sweat. As with any of the exercises I've mentioned, the important thing with an aerobic style of yoga is to find a qualifed teacher who will evaluate your medical condition and adapt the practice to your needs. The style of yoga I advocate for people in recovery, and practice myself, is a slow, gentle and healing practice. It is not an aerobic yoga but does complement other aerobic activites.

Whatever form of exercise you choose, remember to take it easy. The greatest danger facing recovering people who get into exercise is the tendency to be compulsive. You don't have to exercise for three hours straight the first time you go to the gym. Injuries often occur from trying to do too much, too quickly. Take exercise slowly and realize that the benefits are cumulative. A little bit each day goes a long way.

Practicing Hatha yoga is the perfect complement to any cardiovascular exercise you choose. If you follow the yoga approach to exercise, maintain a healthy diet, and allow your body plenty of rest you will enjoy good health and physical vitality.

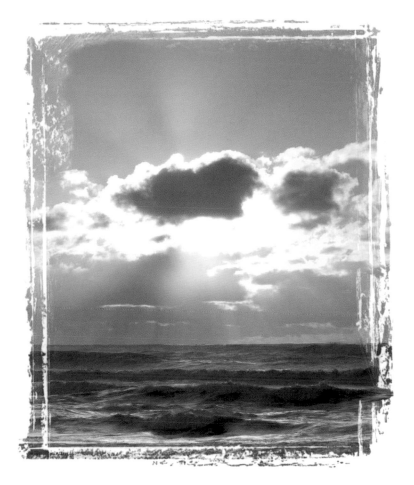

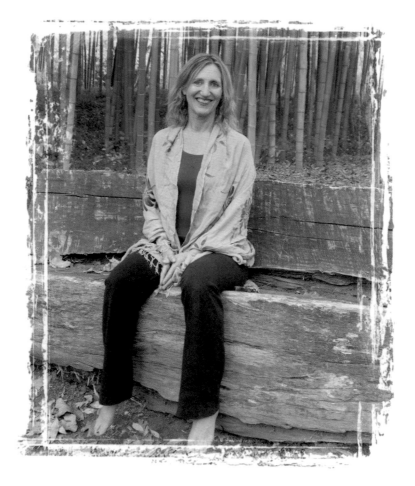

But for the Grace of God.

Recovery is a Lifetime Journey

It took me a long time to understand that life is not about "getting there" but rather about the beauty of the journey itself. This concept is easy to grasp when things are going well for me, but when things aren't happening the way I would like and I'm feeling overwhelmed by the stress of life's situations, I find myself wanting to "fix things" or to be somewhere else or someone else. At these times I have to step back and remind myself that I am powerless over the situation and that my life has become unmanageable. So often in life I come back to the first step. Then I am able to turn it over to my Higher Power and this allows me to accept myself as I am and where I am, without having to control things or run away.

One of the nicest things about 12-Step meetings is that everyone has the right to be exactly where they are on the journey. Some people are crying. Some people are angry. Some are questioning. Others are surrendered and are happy. And these states change for all of us. Those of us who temporarily have more serenity give support to those of us who temporarily have less. In time the faith does grow as you see the program working in your life. And with faith comes serenity. But there will be falls along the way – they are all part of the journey. The important thing is to keep working the steps one day at a time.

Practicing yoga is very similar. You start where you are with your body and take it slowly one day at a time. The idea is not to become perfect or to compete with others, but rather to develop a routine that works positively for you as part of your recovering lifestyle. As you become familiar with the yoga practices and incorporate them into your life, the benefits you receive will help you to understand that yoga, too, is a lifetime practice. When you practice Hatha yoga, your body is strong and flexible, and you have more energy with less stress. If you stop the routine for a while you will notice the difference: more stiffness, less energy, less flexibility, and more stress.

Developing new habits and opening up to alternative ways of living is not always easy. It takes conscious effort. It takes willingness and patience. Often I approach my yoga practice with the attitude of "just for today." Just for today, I will remember to breathe deeply. Just for today, I will think positively about myself and others. Just for today, I will spend time stretching and exercising my body. Just for today, I will eat nutritious food. Just for today, I will meditate. Just for today, I will allow myself to relax.

And, of course my "just for today's" add up to create a healthy lifestyle in which I am taking care of myself. Some days I do better than others. I don't always treat myself well, but I am learning. I keep working at it because I know that taking care of myself is essential to my recovery and continued growth.

One of the most important benefits of yoga in my recovery is that it helps me achieve a stillness of mind. When my mind is still, I can focus on the present moment rather than worrying about the future or thinking about the past. This is especially valuable to me when I have uncomfortable feelings that I want to push down or avoid. Calming my mind and emotions with Hatha yoga helps me acknowledge and accept my feeling without fear. If I am feeling emotional pain I use my deep breathing to help me surrender rather than resist. If I am feeling physical pain I use the postures to help ease the tensions in my body. Relaxation, prayer, and meditation help me remain open to my Higher Power and maintain my spiritual connectedness to life. Hatha yoga helps me accept grace and flow into my life.

Those of us who are recovering from compulsive or addictive behaviors know that unless we break free of our self-destruction routines we will continue to spiral downward in self-defeating ruts that begin to cave in on us. The only difference between a rut and a grave is its dimensions and the dirt on top. Attending meetings and working the steps can prevent us from killing ourselves. Once we open ourselves up to our Higher Power and reach out to a network of support from other recovering people we begin to understand that we are worthy of healing. This is a crucial understanding. Unless we realize that we are worthy of healing and that we deserve the gifts life has to offer, we may sabotage our recovery. Learning to take care of ourselves in loving positive ways is an expression of our acceptance of worth which helps build and reinforce our self-esteem. Taking care of ourselves is loving ourselves.

Practicing Hatha yoga has helped me to take care of myself. It has helped me to learn to relax, to let go of unnecessary anxiety, to appreciate and respect my body, to calm my mind, and to take time out for me. I view my yoga practice the same way I view my 12-Step recovery work: as an on-going process.

It is a practice which can help me the rest of my life if I stay with it. Yoga is not for everyone. But as a recovering person working a 12-Step program, my experience with practicing Hatha yoga is "keep coming back — it works!"

Journal Entry

Yoga, like recovery, isn't about getting and holding the result. There is no end. It is one's life. Recovery is my life and until I embraced that realization I was always looking to get fixed.

I always thought "marriage will fix me, the perfect job will fix me, the thing outside of myself will fix me. The perfect food, drug, relationship, body image." But through yoga I have experienced a state of acceptance of myself exactly as I am this moment. There is only the present moment, until the next moment, until the next moment. One moment following another: A never ending chain of moments that constitutes my entire existence.

Now I understand that I'm OK where I am today, this moment. The outside stuff will always be there, but it doesn't mean I have to obtain something to be OK. I am enough as I am right now. Life isn't perfect, my yoga isn't perfect, my recovery isn't perfect, but it's mine!

I say this on my knees in complete humility. I am grateful for being imperfect; for the fun in exploring, in feeling, in the process. Yoga is a process. Recovery is a process. Life is a process; and together they work.

Laura *(Recovering Adult Child Addict*
Bulimic Workaholic Perfectionist)

Resources

For Information about 12-Step meetings in your area, look for the listing in your phone book under "Alcoholics Anonymous." Also check your local newspaper for listings of other Self Help programs.

To Help with Recovery

Melody Beattie, *The New Codependency: Help And Guidance For Today's Generation* (Simon & Schuster New York 2009)

Melody Beattie, *Codependent No More* (Hazelden, Center City, Minnesota, 1992)

Melody Beattie, *Beyond Codependency* (Harper/Hazelton, New York, 1989)

Patrick J. Carnes PhD., *Facing The Shadow: Starting Sexual And Relationship Recovery* (Gentle Path Press, Carefree, Arizonia, 2005)

Patrick J. Carnes PhD., *A Gentle Path Through The Twelve Steps* (Hazelden, Center City, Minnesota 1994)

Stephanie Covington PhD., *A Womans Way Through The Twelve Steps Workbook* (Hazelton, Minnesota, 2000)

Jeff Jay and Debra Jay, *Love First: A Family's Guide To Intervention* (Hazelton, Center City, Minnesota, 2008)

Stephanie Covington PhD., *A Womans Journal: Helping Women Recover, Revised Edition* (Jossey-Bass, A Wiley Company, San Francisco, 2008)

Pia Medlody, *Facing Love Addiction* (Harper San Francisco, 1992)

Robin Norwood, *Woman Who Love Too Much* (Pocket Books: A Divsion of Simon & Schuster, New York, 2008)

Linda L. Simmons, *The Everything Guide to Addiction and Recovery* (F& W Publications Company, Avon, Massachusetts, 2008)

Twelve Steps And Twelve Traditions (Alcoholics Anonymous World Services Inc., New York, Fortieth printing 2004)

Yoga

Annalisa Cunningham, *Gentle Yoga For Healing Mind, Body, Spirit* (Sterling Publications, New York, 2003)

Nischala Joy Devi, *The Healing Path Of Yoga* (Three Rivers Press, New York, 2000)

Donna Farhi, *The Breathing Book* (Henry Holt & Company, New York, 1996)

Georg Feuerstein, Ph.D and Larry Payne, Ph.D., *Yoga For Dummies* (Hungry Minds, Inc. New York, 1999)

Suza Francina and Jim Jacobs, *The New Yoga For Healthy Aging: Living Longer, Living Stronger and Loving Every Day* (Health Communications, Inc Deerfield Beach, FL 2007)

Suza Francina, *The New Yoga For People Over 50* (Health Communications, Deerfield Beech FL,1997)

Per Van Houten and Rich McCord, *Yoga Therapy For Headache Relief* (Crystal Clarity Publishers, Nevada City, CA 2003)

Gary Kraftsow, *Yoga For Wellness* (Penguin, New York, 1999)

Judith Lasater, *Relax And Renew: Restful Yoga for Stressful Times* (Rodmell Press, Berkeley, CA, 1995)

Darren Main, *Yoga And The Path Of The Urban Mystic* (Findhorn Press, 2001)

Richard Miller, *Yoga Nidra: The Meditative Heart of Yoga* (2005 Sounds True, Boulder Co 2005)

Richard Rosen, *Yoga for 50 +: Moditifed Poses & Techniques for a safe practice* (Ulysses Press Berkeley, CA 2004)

Erich Schiffman, *The Spirit and Practice of Moving into Stillness* (Pocket Books, New York, 1996)

Swami Shivapremananda, *Yoga For Stress Relief* (Random House, New York: 1997)

Linda Sparrow & Patricia Walden, *The Womans Book Of Yoga & Health* (Shambhala Publications, Boston, MA, 2002)

Rita Trieger, *Yoga Heals Your Back: 10-Minute Routines that End Back and Neck Pain* (Fair winds Press 2005)

—

Meditation and Prayer

Stephan Bodian, *Meditation For Dummies 2nd edition* (Wiley Publishing, Inc. Indianapolis, Indiana 2006)

Larry Dossey, MD., *Prayer Is Good Medicine: How to Reap the Healing Benefits of Prayer* (Harper San Francisco,1996)

David Fontana, *Ph.D., Learn To Meditate: A Practical Guide to Self-Discovery and Fulfillment* (Chronicle Books, San Francisco, 1999)

Dharma Singh Khalsa, *Meditation As Medicine: Activate the Power of Your Natural Healing Force* (Fireside of Simon & Schuster Inc., New York 2002)

Jack Kornfield, *Meditation For Beginners* (Sounds True, Inc. Boulder CO, 2008)

Sandra Kynes, *Your Altar: Creating a Sacred Space for Prayer and Meditation* (Llewellyn Publications, Woodbury, MN 2007)

Julie T. Lusk, *Yoga Meditations:Timeless Mind-Body Practices for Awakening* (Whole Person Associates Duluth, MN, 2005)

Darren Main, *The Findhorn Book Of Meditation* (Findhorn Press, 2003)

Doriel Hall, *Discover Meditation* (Ulysses Press, Berkeley CA, 1997)

Maggie Oman Shannon, *Prayers for Hope and Comfort: Reflections, Meditations and Inspirations* (Conari Press, San Francisco, CA 2008)

Geno W. and William G. Borchert, *Wisdom sought through Prayer and Mediation* (from the Sunday 11th Step Meetings at the Wolfe Street Center in Little Rock Hazelden, Center City Minnesota 2008)

Diet and Health

Prescription For Nutritional Healing: The A to Z Guide to Supplements, 4th edition (Penguin Putman Inc. New York, NY 2006)

Blanche Agassy, *Global Kitchen: Vegetarian Favorites from The Expanding Light Retreat* (McCord Crystal Clarity Publishers, Nevada City CA, 2002)

Todd Dacey with Jia Patton, *Vegan Inspiration Whole Food Recipes for Life* (Blue Dophin Publishing, Inc. Nevada City CA 2008)

Dharma Singh Khalsa MD, *Food As Medicine* (Atria Books, New York 2003)

Nancy Mair, *The Intimate Vegetarian {a cookbook}* (Crystal Clarity Publishers, Nevada City CA, 2000)

Wendy North, *The Raw Transformation Energizing your Life with Living Foods* (Atlantic Books, Berkeley, CA 2006)

Dr. Dean Ornish, *Everyday Cooking: 150 Easy, Low Fat, High Flavor Recipes* (Harper Collins, New York,1997)

Steve Petusevsky and Whole Foods Market Team Members, *The Whole Foods Market Cookbook - A Guide to Natural Foods with 350 Recipies* (Clarkson Potter Publishers New York, NY 2002)

Kay Lynne Sherman, *The Findhorn Book of Vegetarian Recipes* (Findhorn Press, 2003)

Sivananda Yoga Center, *The Yoga Cookbook: Vegetarian Food for Body and Mind* (Fireside New York, NY 1999)

Faith Stone and Rachael Guidry, *Yoga Ktichen: Recipes from the Shoshoni Yoga Retreat* (The Book Publishing Co, Summertown TN 2004)

Andrew Weil, *Natural Health, Natural Medicine - The complete Guide to wellness and Self Care for Optimum Health* (Houghton Mifflin Co. New York, NY 2004)

To order Annalisa's *"Stretch & Surrender"* CD, please go to:
www.openingheartjourneys.com/cds.html
or email: info@openingheartjourneys.com
or call: 530-343-9944 (USA)

To consult the complete Findhorn Press List, please visit:
www.findhornpress.com

For information on the Findhorn Foundation Community:
www.findhorn.org

FINDHORN PRESS

Life changing books

For a complete catalogue,
please contact:

Findhorn Press Ltd
305a The Park, Findhorn
Forres IV36 3TE
Scotland, UK

Telephone
+44-(0)1309-690582
Fax
+44-(0)131-777-2711
eMail
info@findhornpress.com

or consult our catalogue online
(with secure order facility) on
www.findhornpress.com

For information on the Findhorn Foundation:
www.findhorn.org